Advancements in Individualized Plastic and Reconstructive Surgery

Advancements in Individualized Plastic and Reconstructive Surgery

Guest Editors

Paul Immanuel Heidekrueger
Peter Niclas Broer
Denis C. Ehrl

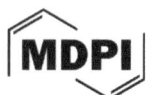

Basel • Beijing • Wuhan • Barcelona • Belgrade • Novi Sad • Cluj • Manchester

Guest Editors

Paul Immanuel Heidekrueger
Centre of Plastic, Aesthetic,
Hand and
Reconstructive Surgery
University of Regensburg
Regensburg
Germany

Peter Niclas Broer
Department of Plastic,
Reconstructive, Hand and
Burn Surgery
Bogenhausen Academic
Teaching Hospital Munich
Munich
Germany

Denis C. Ehrl
Department of Plastic,
Reconstructive and
Hand Surgery
University Hospital of the
Paracelsus Medical University
Nuremberg
Germany

Editorial Office
MDPI AG
Grosspeteranlage 5
4052 Basel, Switzerland

This is a reprint of the Special Issue, published open access by the journal *Journal of Clinical Medicine* (ISSN 2077-0383), freely accessible at: https://www.mdpi.com/journal/jcm/special_issues/T1J22KIEEO.

For citation purposes, cite each article independently as indicated on the article page online and as indicated below:

Lastname, A.A.; Lastname, B.B. Article Title. *Journal Name* **Year**, *Volume Number*, Page Range.

ISBN 978-3-7258-4409-8 (Hbk)
ISBN 978-3-7258-4410-4 (PDF)
https://doi.org/10.3390/books978-3-7258-4410-4

© 2025 by the authors. Articles in this book are Open Access and distributed under the Creative Commons Attribution (CC BY) license. The book as a whole is distributed by MDPI under the terms and conditions of the Creative Commons Attribution-NonCommercial-NoDerivs (CC BY-NC-ND) license (https://creativecommons.org/licenses/by-nc-nd/4.0/).

Contents

Denis Ehrl, Paul I. Heidekrueger, Riccardo E. Giunta and Nikolaus Wachtel
Giant Penoscrotal Lymphedema—What to Do? Presentation of a Curative Treatment Algorithm
Reprinted from: *J. Clin. Med.* **2023**, *12*, 7586, https://doi.org/10.3390/jcm12247586 1

Hsiu-Hsia Lin, Jyun-Cheng Kuo, Lun-Jou Lo and Cheng-Ting Ho
Optimizing Orthognathic Surgery: Leveraging the Average Skull as a Dynamic Template for Surgical Simulation and Planning in 30 Patient Cases
Reprinted from: *J. Clin. Med.* **2023**, *12*, 7758, https://doi.org/10.3390/jcm12247758 11

Julius M. Mayer, Sophie I. Spies, Carla K. Mayer, Cédric Zubler, Rafael Loucas and Thomas Holzbach
How to Treat a Cyclist's Nodule?—Introduction of a Novel, ICG-Assisted Approach
Reprinted from: *J. Clin. Med.* **2024**, *13*, 1124, https://doi.org/10.3390/jcm13041124 22

Angela Augustin, Ines Schoberleitner, Sophie-Marie Unterhumer, Johanna Krapf, Thomas Bauer and Dolores Wolfram
PlasmaBlade versus Electrocautery for Deep Inferior Epigastric Perforator Flap Harvesting in Autologous Breast Reconstruction: A Comparative Clinical Outcome Study
Reprinted from: *J. Clin. Med.* **2024**, *13*, 2388, https://doi.org/10.3390/jcm13082388 32

Tonatiuh Flores, Celina Kerschbaumer, Florian J. Jaklin, Christina Glisic, Hugo Sabitzer, Jakob Nedomansky, et al.
High-Volume Liposuction in Lipedema Patients: Effects on Serum Vitamin D
Reprinted from: *J. Clin. Med.* **2024**, *13*, 2846, https://doi.org/10.3390/jcm13102846 45

Daihun Kang
Advancing Fingertip Regeneration: Outcomes from a New Conservative Treatment Protocol
Reprinted from: *J. Clin. Med.* **2024**, *13*, 3646, https://doi.org/10.3390/jcm13133646 57

Alicia Dean, Orlando Estévez, Concepción Centella, Alba Sanjuan-Sanjuan, Marina E. Sánchez-Frías and Francisco J. Alamillos
Surgical Navigation and CAD-CAM-Designed PEEK Prosthesis for the Surgical Treatment of Facial Intraosseous Vascular Anomalies
Reprinted from: *J. Clin. Med.* **2024**, *13*, 4602, https://doi.org/10.3390/jcm13164602 70

Asja T. Malsagova, Amin El-Habbassi, Moritz Billner, Maresa Berns, Tamas Pueski, Karl J. Bodenschatz, et al.
Long-Term Functional Outcomes Following Enzymatic Debridement of Deep Hand Burns Using Nexobrid®: A Retrospective Analysis
Reprinted from: *J. Clin. Med.* **2024**, *13*, 4729, https://doi.org/10.3390/jcm13164729 89

Guadalupe Santamaría Salvador, Esteban Acosta Muñoz, Juan Samaniego Rojas, Charles Hidalgo Quishpe, Juan S. Izquierdo-Condoy, Jorge Vasconez-Gonzalez and Esteban Ortiz-Prado
Flap-Free Tendon Coverage Using Autologous Fat Grafts Enhanced with Platelet-Rich Plasma and Growth Factors at a Secondary Level Hospital: A Case Report
Reprinted from: *J. Clin. Med.* **2024**, *13*, 5640, https://doi.org/10.3390/jcm13185640 100

Tonatiuh Flores, Barbara Kremsner, Jana Schön, Julia Riedl, Hugo Sabitzer, Christina Glisic, et al.
Lipedema: Complications in High-Volume Liposuction Are Linked to Preoperative Anemia
Reprinted from: *J. Clin. Med.* **2024**, *13*, 7779, https://doi.org/10.3390/jcm13247779 109

Tonatiuh Flores, Florian J. Jaklin, Martin S. Mayrl, Celina Kerschbaumer, Christina Glisic, Kristina Pfoser, et al.
Paravertebral Blocks in Implant-Based Breast Reconstruction Do Not Induce Increased Postoperative Blood or Drainage Fluid Loss
Reprinted from: *J. Clin. Med.* **2025**, *14*, 1832, https://doi.org/10.3390/jcm14061832 . . . . **123**

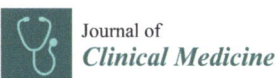

Article

Giant Penoscrotal Lymphedema—What to Do? Presentation of a Curative Treatment Algorithm

Denis Ehrl [1,*], Paul I. Heidekrueger [2], Riccardo E. Giunta [1] and Nikolaus Wachtel [1]

1. Division of Hand, Plastic and Aesthetic Surgery, University Hospital, LMU Munich, 80336 Munich, Germany
2. Centre of Plastic, Aesthetic, Hand and Reconstructive Surgery, University of Regensburg, 93053 Regensburg, Germany
* Correspondence: denis.ehrl@med.uni-muenchen.de

Abstract: Background: While rare, penoscrotal lymphedema (PL) is accompanied with devastating effects on the quality of life of patients. Moreover, especially for patients with excessive (giant) PL, no standardized curative treatment has been defined. This article therefore retrospectively evaluates the authors' surgical treatment approach for giant PL, which includes resection alone or in combination with a free vascularized lymph node transfer (VLNT). Methods: A total of ten patients met the inclusion criteria. One patient dropped out of the study before therapy commenced. Eight of the nine remaining patients presented with end-stage (giant) PL. One patient presented with manifest pitting edema. All patients were treated with penoscrotal resection and reconstruction. Additionally, five patients received VLNT into the groin or scrotum. Results: The extent of the lymphedema was specified with a treatment-oriented classification system. The median follow-up was 49.0 months. No patient showed a recurrence. Patients who received VLNT into the scrotum displayed a significantly improved lymphatic transport of the scrotum. Conclusions: Advanced PL should be treated in a standardized surgical fashion as suggested by our proposed algorithm. VLNT from the lateral thoracic region into the scrotum must be considered. If treated correctly, surgical intervention of end-stage PL leads to good results with a low recurrence rate.

Keywords: penoscrotal lymphedema; free vascularized lymph node transfer; lymphedema

1. Introduction

While rare, penoscrotal lymphedema (PL) is typically endemic to Africa and Asia and is caused by lymphatic obstruction due to filariasis (typically Wuscheria bancrofti) or bacterial infection [1–4]. Other secondary causes include tumors, lymphadenectomy, radiotherapy, or disorders of the fluid balance, such as heart or kidney disease. Rarely, the edema can present as a symptom of a primary lymphatic malformations (i.e., Meigs and Milroy's disease) [5–7]. Moreover, during the last two decades, an increasing number of articles have reported of cases with no clear etiology, termed idiopathic penoscrotal lymphedema (IPL) [5,8].

While benign, PL is accompanied with devastating effects on social life, sexual function, and hygiene [1,8,9]. First-line therapy for bacterial-associated PL is antibiotic treatment [10]. However, other etiologies regularly require surgery [5,8,11]. Here, primary closure, coverage with skin grafts, flap reconstruction, and microsurgical lymphaticovenous anastomoses (LVAs) in combination with surgical resection have been described [1,11–13]. Interestingly, while promising for other cases of lymphedema [8,14,15], vascularized lymph node transfer (VLNT) has not yet been assessed as a treatment for PL and was only described in two cases of PL with transplantation to the groin (17). Moreover, due to the rarity of the pathology to date, no clear consensus has been presented regarding diagnostics and, in particular, standardized treatment [4]. The purpose of this retrospective case series was therefore to evaluate the authors' treatment approach for PL, which includes scrotal and penile resection and subsequent reconstruction alone or in combination with a free VLNT. Additionally, we set out to evaluate and present a new classification of PL and to define an algorithmic approach for the surgical treatment of PL. For this, we analyzed surgical and functional outcomes of scrotal and penile reconstructions without or with VLNT to suggest the best therapeutic option for PL.

2. Materials and Methods

2.1. Patient Selection/Inclusion Criteria

The clinical charts of all patients who presented with PL and received surgery were retrospectively reviewed from 2018 to 2022. The first patient reviewed presented with a gigantic IPL and therefore was published in 2018 [13]. Subsequently, patients with PL, both primary (idiopathic) and due to secondary causes, were transferred to our department on a regular basis. Indication for surgical therapy was an end-stage PL (stage III), according to the consensus statement of the International Lymphology Conference of 2020, or a failure of complete decongestive therapy [16]. Both primary (idiopathic) and secondary PL were included in this study. Any type of surgical procedure was included (scrotectomy/penile lymphedema reduction and/or VLNT). A chart review was performed to obtain a possible etiology, including serological and hematological laboratory tests to exclude parasite as well as bacterial infection. Moreover, charts were assessed for pre- and postoperative diagnostics, such as lymphoscintigraphy and/or MRI. Outcome parameters included postoperative complications, including surgical site infection, erectile dysfunction, donor site morbidity, and recurrence of lymphedema. The extent of recurrence was classified according to the consensus statement on the diagnosis and treatment of peripheral lymphedema of the International Lymphology Conference of 2020, where stage I (swelling and fluid accumulation) is classified as minor, stage II (manifest pitting edema) as moderate, and stage III (lymphostatic elephantiasis) as major recurrence [16]. Patients presenting with varicocele were not included in the study.

2.2. Scrotal and Penile Surgery

Scrotal resection (scrotectomy) and reconstruction was described in detail previously [1,3,13]. In accordance with our classification (Table 1), whenever the lymphedema affected the penis, resection of penile skin and subcutaneous tissue was performed. In case of mild to advanced PL, the penile skin is reconstructed using split skin grafts. For patients with advanced PL (buried penis), the penile skin is reconstructed with a dorsal flap from the mons pubis (wrap-around technique) [13]. In all patients, the excised tissue was sent for histological assessment.

Table 1. Treatment-oriented classification of penoscrotal lymphedema.

Stage	Criteria	Number of Patients
I	Isolated Lymphedema of the Scrotum	2
II	Combined Lymphedema of the Scrotum and Penis	4
III	Combined Lymphedema of the Scrotum and Penis and Buried Penis	3

2.3. Vascularized Lymph Node Transfer

For all patients with VLNT, CT angiography was performed preoperatively to assess donor as well as recipient vessels for transfer. The lymph nodes were harvested from the lateral thoracic region and axilla (anterior axillary lymph nodes/level 2). The lateral thoracic artery and vein were used as nutrient vessels. Additionally, a skin island was harvested to allow for adequate monitoring after microsurgical transfer. Initially, for patients 5 to 7, vascularized lymph nodes were transferred into the groin with arterial and venous anastomosis to the superficial circumflex iliac vessels, as described previously [17].

However, this approach does not correspond to the primary physiological lymph drainage from the scrotum. For this reason, we modified this approach in two patients (patient 8 and 9), such that vascularized lymph nodes were (corresponding to the primary physiological lymph drainage) transferred directly into the scrotum with the superficial external pudendal artery and vein as recipient vessels [18]. Microsurgical arterial and venous anastomoses were performed in standard fashion. Monitoring was performed with clinical and regular Doppler ultrasound control as well as using an Oxygen to See (O2C, LEA Medizintechnik, Gießen, Germany) device for continuous monitoring [19].

3. Results

A total of ten patients met the inclusion criteria (Figure 1). The patients had a mean age of 41.7 years (24 to 59 years) at surgery. One patient dropped out of the study before surgical therapy commenced due to the fact that he presented with massive obesity (BMI of 52) and planned to lose weight and subsequently be treated with an abdominoplasty as well as penoscrotal reconstruction in combination with free VLNT. However, due to severe local infection, his scrotum and penis were amputated in another hospital.

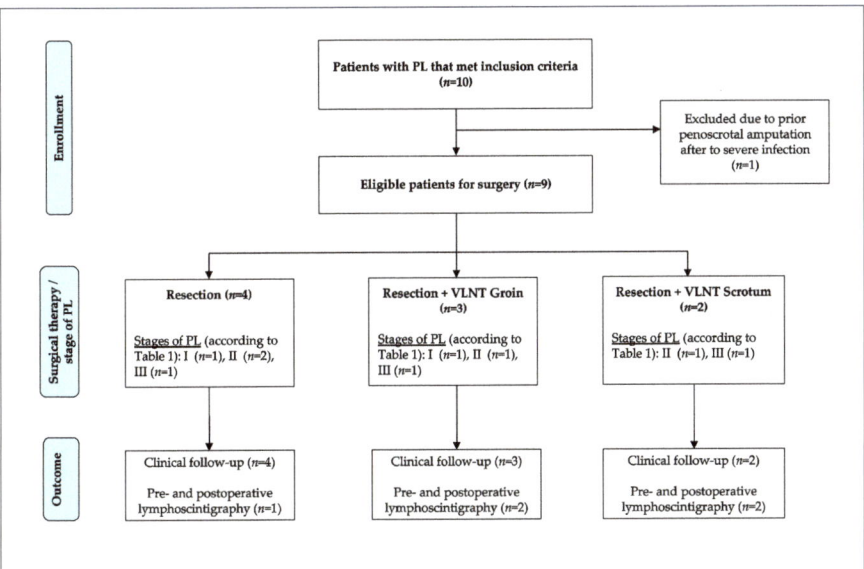

Figure 1. Study flow diagram. Nine patients were eligible for surgical therapy of penoscrotal lymphedema (PL). Eight of these patients presented with end-stage penoscrotal lymphedema (PL) (lymphostatic elephantiasis) and one patient presented with a manifest pitting edema [16]. The extent of the lymphedema was further specified with a treatment-oriented grading system (see also Table 1). All patients received scrotal and penile resection surgery in a single-stage procedure, with or without vascularized lymph node transfer (VLNT) into the groin or scrotum.

Seven of the nine remaining patients presented with combined PL, and two patients presented with scrotal lymphedema only. Nearly all (eight out of nine) patients presented with stage III lymphedema (according to the consensus statement of the International Lymphology Conference of 2020, i.e., lymphostatic elephantiasis), while one patient presented with stage II lymphedema after failure of complete decongestive therapy, [16]. These all met the inclusion criteria for surgical therapy. As all patients were transferred to our department after extensive conservative treatment and/or with end-stage PL, no patient was treated with non-surgical options.

The extent of the lymphedema was further specified with a treatment-oriented classification system that was developed at our department (Table 1). An overview of the study cohort can be found in Table 2.

Table 2. Overview of the surgical procedures performed in the study cohort. Eight patients presented with end-stage penoscrotal lymphedema (PL) (lymphostatic elephantiasis), and patient 7 presented with a manifest pitting edema [16]. The extent of the lymphedema was further specified with a treatment-oriented grading system (Table 1). For all patients, scrotal and penile resection and subsequent reconstruction alone, combined with vascularized lymph node transfer into the groin (VLNT Groin), or combined with vascularized lymph node transfer into the scrotum (VLNT Scrotum) was performed. All patients were treated in a single-stage procedure.

Patient	Etiology	Treatment-Oriented Stage of PL	Surgical Procedure	Follow-Up Period (Months)
1	Primary	III	Resection	67
2	Primary	I	Resection	59
3	Secondary	II	Resection	52
4	Primary	II	Resection	45
5	Primary	II	Resection + VLNT Groin	58
6	Secondary	III	Resection + VLNT Groin	49
7	Primary	I	Resection + VLNT Groin	37
8	Primary	III	Resection + VLNT Scrotum	18
9	Primary	II	Resection + VLNT Scrotum	16

Seven patients presented with primary (idiopathic) and two with secondary PL (resection of the sigmoid colon due to diverticulitis (patient 3) and treatment for anal carcinoma, which included surgery and radiation therapy (patient 6)). All patients received scrotal and penile resection surgery in a single-stage procedure, with or without VLNT (Table 2).

The lymphedema of seven patients were preoperatively assessed with lymphoscintigraphy. One patient was assessed with an MRI scan, and one patient had no preoperative imaging of his PL. Preoperative diagnostic imagining for the eight patients showed none (three), minor (one), moderate (two), or severe (two) local impairment of scrotal lymphatic transport. One patient with moderate impairment of scrotal lymphatic transport also demonstrated a reduced lymphatic transport of the adjacent lower extremity (patient 6, secondary lymphedema after treatment for anal carcinoma).

The median follow-up was 49.0 months (16 to 67 months). All nine patients showed no recurrence in this period. However, one patient presented with a hydrocele testis during follow-up. He initially presented with a combined lymphedema of the scrotum and a buried penis (patient 6, also refer to Table 2) as well as lymphedema of both lower extremities after treatment for anal carcinoma and was initially treated with surgical resection of penile skin and subcutaneous tissue as well as VLNT to the groin.

Five patients (patients 2, 6, 7, 8, and 9) received postoperative lymphoscintigraphy. The postoperative lymphoscintigraphy of patients 2 and 7 demonstrated no significant change when compared to the preoperative findings (lymphoscintigraphy was taken five and four months after surgery, respectively). Postoperative lymphoscintigraphy (32 months after surgery) of patient 6 (scrotal and penile resection followed by VLNT into the groin) similarly showed no significant change in the scrotal lymph transport. Interestingly, a significant improvement in the lymphedema of the ipsilateral leg after VLNT into the groin was observed in this patient, while the lymphatic transport was unchanged in the contralateral leg.

Postoperative lymphoscintigraphy of patients who received VLNT into the scrotum (patients 8 and 9), however, showed significantly improved lymphatic transport of the scrotum three and four months after surgical intervention (scrotal and penile resection combined with VLNT into the scrotum).

For patients with vascularized lymph node transfer, no donor site morbidity on the trunk was observed. Additionally, no complications at the penoscrotal surgical site were observed. Histologic examination for all patients showed chronic lymphostasis, surrounded by fibrous tissue.

4. Discussion

Filarial infection with Wuscheria bancrofti, Brugia malayi or timori represents the most common etiology for lymphedema worldwide [4,5,20]. Consequently, most cases of PL are caused by this infection [4,5]. However, in regions where filarial worms are rarely found, such as Europe, Northern America, and Australia, other etiologies cause the majority of PL. Moreover, a growing number of idiopathic cases in these regions have been described previously [5,8,11]. Our study confirms these findings, as none of the patients showed filarial infection and only two presented with secondary PL. The other patients were classified as primary (idiopathic) PL (Table 2). Considering the excessive dimensions of the majority of lymphedema presented in this study and/or poor efficacy of previous long-term conservative treatment options, all patients received surgical treatment (Figures 2–4) [4,8].

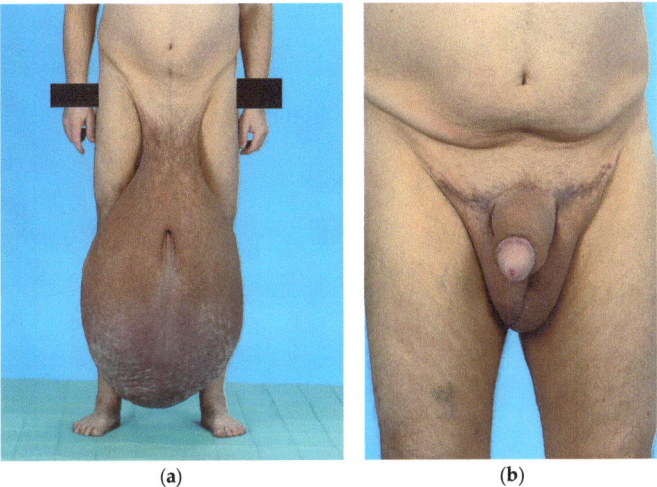

Figure 2. (a) Patient 1 with giant stage III penoscrotal lymphedema (PL), according to the classification in Table 1, before treatment and (b) 6 weeks after surgery (resection and flap reconstruction of scrotum and penis).

PL is a rare pathology, and a reduced number of patients is therefore to be expected [4]. Nevertheless, the present study encompasses one of the largest collections of clinical cases of advanced PL. While two other studies included more patients in total, the authors of both studies recruited a majority of patients with early-stage PL, where no or only minor surgical intervention (i.e., circumcision) was necessary [4,8]. Moreover, when assessing previous classifications of PL, we found these focus predominantly on etiologic or morphologic aspects [5,8]. In the current study, the extent of the PL was therefore further specified with a new classification (Table 1) [16]. Importantly, here, we grade PL according to the subsequent surgical procedure necessary for treatment.

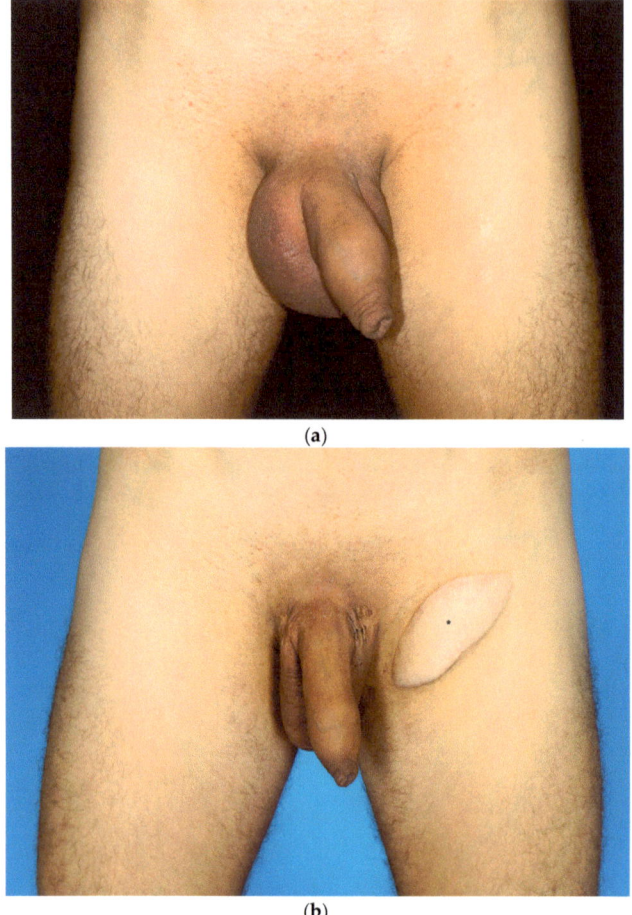

Figure 3. (**a**) Patient 7 with isolated lymphedema of the scrotum (stage I PL according to the classification in Table 1) before treatment and (**b**) 27 months after surgery (resection and flap reconstruction of scrotum combined with a vascularized lymph node transfer (VLNT) into the groin). The monitoring island of the VLNT in (**b**) is marked with an asterisk.

Guiotto and colleagues thoroughly reviewed the previously published surgical treatment options for the therapy of PL [11]. The authors identified three surgical techniques, where two groups represent palliative treatment concepts: surgical resection and primary closure, or skin graft and resection followed by reconstruction with local flaps. A third group with curative intent was identified. Here, resection was followed by microsurgical LVA to improve lymphatic flow in the penoscrotal area. Interestingly, to date, only Phan et al. have reported two cases of VLNT to the groin for the treatment of PL [17]. This is in contrast with promising data on LVA and, in particular, VLNT for other advanced types of lymphedema [14,21,22]. Indeed, while LVA seems to be more effective in earlier stages of lymphedema, lymphatic vessels become sclerotic in more advanced stages, making VLNT the better option for advanced PL [11,14]. Therefore, while treating advanced PL, we introduced VLNT as therapeutic treatment for PL.

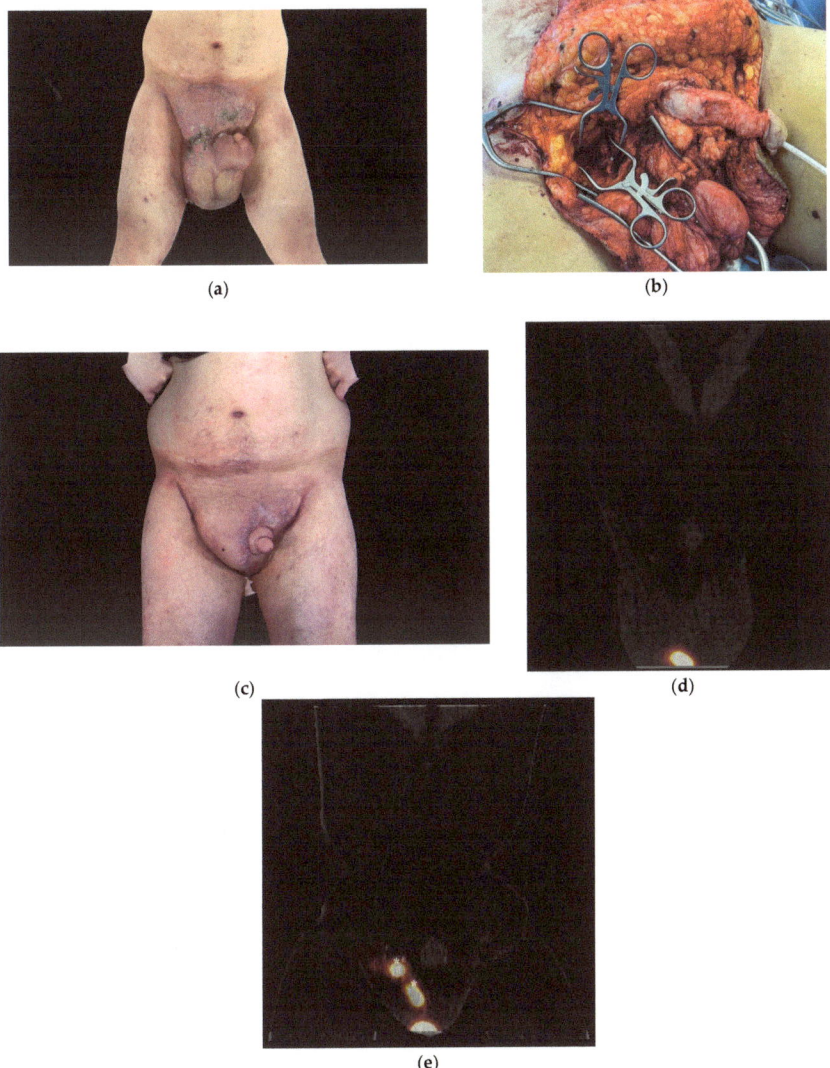

Figure 4. Images of advanced stage III penoscrotal lymphedema (PL), according to the classification in Table 1, (patient 8) (**a**) before treatment, (**b**) during surgery, and (**c**) after treatment. Panels (**d**,**e**) show low-dose SPECT-CT scans, before and after surgery. At initial presentation, the patient suffered from severe local infection and folliculitis and was therefore treated with long-term antibiotics (**a**). Surgery included resection and flap reconstruction of scrotum and penis combined with a vascularized lymph node transfer (VLNT) into the scrotum (**b**), with the superficial external pudendal artery and vein as recipient vessels (marked with an asterisk). Panel (**c**) shows the result 8 months after surgery. The monitoring island of the VLNT in (**c**) is marked with an asterisk. The skin and subcutaneous tissue of the island may be removed 6 months after surgery to further reduce the volume of the newly fabricated scrotum. Lymphoscintigraphy, including low-dose SPECT-CT scans, showed significantly improved lymphatic transport of the scrotum 3 months after surgical intervention (**e**), when compared to preoperative findings (**d**). The transplanted lymph nodes in (**e**) are marked with an asterisk.

Anatomically, the first lymphatic drainage of the subcutaneous tissue and skin of the scrotum, as well as penis, is via the medial group of the superficial inguinal lymph nodes [11]. A previous publication describes lymph node transfer into the groin for the treatment of PL [17]. It is unclear, however, if a vascularized lymph node transfer into the groin only improves lymphatic drainage of the ipsilateral lower limb and if the combined resection of PL alone is responsible for the results observed by us and others. Moreover, it seems logical to transfer the lymph node into the anatomically affected area, i.e., the scrotum, thereby increasing the likelihood of improved lymphatic drainage. During our study, we therefore altered the VLNT from the groin to the scrotum.

Our clinical experience as well as the findings of the current literature led to the development of an algorithm where we propose a therapeutic protocol with the intent for curative treatment of advanced PL (Figure 5). In our opinion, standardized resection, flap reconstruction, and/or skin grafting (for the penile body at stage II PL, also see Table 1) in combination with VLNT into the scrotum seems to be the best option for a curative treatment for advanced PL. Indeed, similar protocols have been previously proposed for the treatment of upper and lower extremity lymphedema with good long-term results [23–25]. These demonstrate the beneficial effect of a combined therapeutic approach of reductive and microsurgical procedures for the treatment of lymphedema. The resection of tissue reduces the increased solid tissue component (predominantly fibroadipose tissue as well as proinflammatory cytokines), leading to a decrease in overall lymphatic load. Microsurgical procedures, such as VLNT and LVA, effectively improve the lymphatic transport and thereby prevent a re-accumulation of lymphatic fluid in the affected region [23,25].

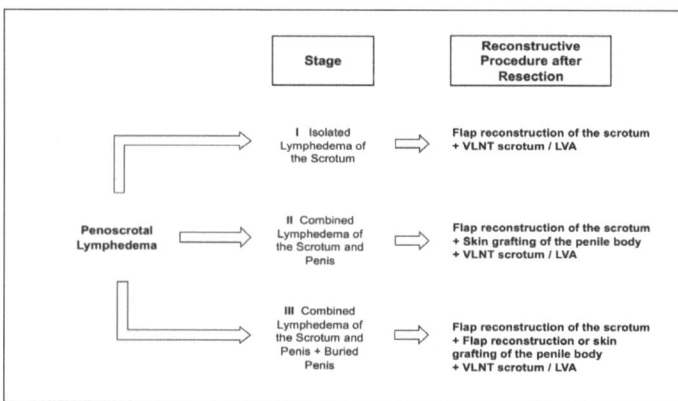

Figure 5. Proposed therapeutic algorithm for the treatment of penoscrotal lymphedema (PL) (according to the proposed treatment-oriented classification presented in Table 1). Prior to any surgical intervention, all conservative treatment options must have been pursued. If these fail, the following surgical options should be considered according to the stage of PL. For resection, standardized incisions should be performed as described previously by us and others [1,3,13]. Reconstruction of the scrotum can then be performed using flaps containing excess skin and subcutaneous tissue from the medial thigh (**stage I PL**). At **stage II PL**, reconstruction of the penile body is best accomplished with skin grafting. Due to the extensive skin excess around the mons pubis in **stage III PL**, sufficient healthy skin and subcutaneous tissue is available for flap reconstruction of the penile body in most cases. If flap reconstruction is not possible due to poor quality of tissue, we recommend skin grafting of the penile body (i.e., analogous to stage II PL). In combination with scrotal and penile reconstruction, we recommend a vascularized lymph node transfer (VLNT) directly into the anatomically affected area of the scrotum, thereby increasing the likelihood of improved lymphatic drainage. Alternatively, lymphaticovenous anastomoses (LVA) can be performed.

In the present study, no patient demonstrated with a recurrence, regardless of whether a VLNT was performed or not (Table 2). Nevertheless, the postoperative lymphoscintigraphy of patients with VLNT into the scrotum showed significantly improved lymphatic transport (patients 8 and 9), while the lymphoscintigraphy of patients who received no VLNT or a VLNT into the groin (patients 2, 6, and 7) was unchanged for the scrotum. Interestingly, patient 6 presented an improved lymphatic transport of the ipsilateral leg after receiving a VLNT into the groin. These findings therefore support our proposed treatment algorithm for PL, as they suggest an advantage of a VLNT into the scrotum, as opposed to no transfer or a transfer into the groin.

However, our conclusions remain suggestive as our study encompasses a limited number of cases as well as three different therapeutic approaches in an already small study population (resection alone and in combination with a VLNT into the groin or the scrotum). This is a clear limitation of our study. Moreover, our suggested algorithm is predominantly based on our clinical experience as well as similar protocols that were presented previously for other areas affected by chronic lymphedema (Figure 5) [23,25]. Thus, large-scale multicentric studies, with a prospective and randomized study design, are warranted. These would overcome the limitations caused by the low overall incidence of PL. A future study design should include a prospective assessment of the possible benefit of VLNT into the scrotum to effectively treat PL. Additionally, our study lacks objective outcome measurements for the quality of life as well as aesthetic aspects. While it seems highly plausible that these parameters are improved after treatment (Figures 2 and 4), the lack of an objective assessment of these is a limitation of this study.

5. Conclusions

End-stage PL, although rare, should be treated in a standardized surgical fashion. VLNT from the lateral thoracic region into the scrotum must be considered as the donor-site morbidity is low and it seems highly likely that this procedure offers a curative treatment option. If treated correctly, surgical intervention of end-stage PL (lymphostatic elephantiasis) results in good outcomes with a low recurrence rate (Figures 2 and 4). Moreover, moderate PL with pitting edema may also be successfully treated with the proposed surgical technique (Figure 3).

Author Contributions: Conceptualization, D.E., P.I.H., R.E.G. and N.W.; Data curation, N.W.; Formal analysis, D.E., P.I.H., R.E.G. and N.W.; Investigation, D.E., P.I.H. and N.W.; Methodology, R.E.G. and N.W.; Project administration, D.E.; Resources, D.E., P.I.H. and N.W.; Software, N.W.; Supervision, D.E.; Validation, D.E., P.I.H., R.E.G. and N.W.; Visualization, N.W.; Writing—original draft, D.E. and N.W.; Writing—review and editing, D.E., P.I.H., R.E.G. and N.W. All authors have read and agreed to the published version of the manuscript.

Funding: This research received no external funding.

Institutional Review Board Statement: Informed consent was obtained from all patients involved in this study. Approval for the study was granted by the regional medical ethics committee (21-0475, LMU Munich, Germany). Moreover, this study was conducted in accordance with the principles set forth in the Helsinki Declaration.

Informed Consent Statement: Informed consent has been obtained from the patients to publish this paper.

Data Availability Statement: The data presented in this study are available on request from the corresponding author. The data are not publicly available due to privacy concerns of the patients enrolled in this study.

Acknowledgments: We would like to thank Hans Schmid, of the Department of Nuclear Medicine, LMU Munich, for providing excellent lymphoscintigraphic images.

Conflicts of Interest: The authors declare no conflict of interest.

References

1. Brotherhood, H.L.; Metcalfe, M.; Goldenberg, L.; Pommerville, P.; Bowman, C.; Naysmith, D. A surgical challenge: Idiopathic scrotal elephantiasis. *Can. Urol. Assoc. J.* **2014**, *8*, E500–E507. [CrossRef]
2. Yonder, S.; Pandey, J. Filarial Hydrocele. In *StatPearls*; StatPearls Publishing LLC.: Treasure Island, FL, USA, 2022.
3. Hornberger, B.J.; Elmore, J.M.; Roehrborn, C.G. Idiopathic scrotal elephantiasis. *Urology* **2005**, *65*, 389. [CrossRef] [PubMed]
4. Kaciulyte, J.; Garutti, L.; Spadoni, D.; Velazquez-Mujica, J.; Losco, L.; Ciudad, P.; Marcasciano, M.; Lo Torto, F.; Casella, D.; Ribuffo, D.; et al. Genital Lymphedema and How to Deal with It: Pearls and Pitfalls from over 38 Years of Experience with Unusual Lymphatic System Impairment. *Medicina* **2021**, *57*, 1175. [CrossRef]
5. McDougal, W.S. Lymphedema of the external genitalia. *J. Urol.* **2003**, *170*, 711–716. [CrossRef]
6. Connell, F.C.; Gordon, K.; Brice, G.; Keeley, V.; Jeffery, S.; Mortimer, P.S.; Mansour, S.; Ostergaard, P. The classification and diagnostic algorithm for primary lymphatic dysplasia: An update from 2010 to include molecular findings. *Clin. Genet.* **2013**, *84*, 303–314. [CrossRef]
7. Connell, F.; Brice, G.; Jeffery, S.; Keeley, V.; Mortimer, P.; Mansour, S. A new classification system for primary lymphatic dysplasias based on phenotype. *Clin. Genet.* **2010**, *77*, 438–452. [CrossRef] [PubMed]
8. Garaffa, G.; Christopher, N.; Ralph, D.J. The management of genital lymphoedema. *BJU Int.* **2008**, *102*, 480–484. [CrossRef] [PubMed]
9. Denzinger, S.; Watzlawek, E.; Burger, M.; Wieland, W.F.; Otto, W. Giant scrotal elephantiasis of inflammatory etiology: A case report. *J. Med. Case Rep.* **2007**, *1*, 23. [CrossRef]
10. Nelson, R.A.; Alberts, G.L.; King, L.E., Jr. Penile and scrotal elephantiasis caused by indolent Chlamydia trachomatis infection. *Urology* **2003**, *61*, 224. [CrossRef]
11. Guiotto, M.; Bramhall, R.J.; Campisi, C.; Raffoul, W.; di Summa, P.G. A Systematic Review of Outcomes after Genital Lymphedema Surgery: Microsurgical Reconstruction Versus Excisional Procedures. *Ann. Plast. Surg.* **2019**, *83*, e85–e91. [CrossRef]
12. Lin, T.; Lin, Y.Z.; Wu, Y.P.; Lin, T.T.; Chen, D.N.; Wei, Y.; Xue, X.Y.; Xu, N. Penoscrotal edema: A case report and literature review. *BMC Urol.* **2019**, *19*, 22. [CrossRef]
13. Ehrl, D.; Tritschler, S.; Haas, E.M.; Alhadlg, A.; Giunta, R.E. Skrotales Lymphödem-Falldarstellung einer skrotalen Elephantiasis inklusive Operationstechnik. *Handchir. Mikrochir. Plast. Chir.* **2018**, *50*, 299–302. [CrossRef] [PubMed]
14. Scaglioni, M.F.; Arvanitakis, M.; Chen, Y.C.; Giovanoli, P.; Chia-Shen Yang, J.; Chang, E.I. Comprehensive review of vascularized lymph node transfers for lymphedema: Outcomes and complications. *Microsurgery* **2016**, *38*, 222–229. [CrossRef] [PubMed]
15. Dionyssiou, D.; Sarafis, A.; Tsimponis, A.; Kalaitzoglou, A.; Arsos, G.; Demiri, E. Long-Term Outcomes of Lymph Node Transfer in Secondary Lymphedema and Its Correlation with Flap Characteristics. *Cancers* **2021**, *13*, 6198. [CrossRef] [PubMed]
16. Executive Committee of the International Society of Lymphology. The diagnosis and treatment of peripheral lymphedema: 2020 Consensus Document of the International Society of Lymphology. *Lymphology* **2020**, *53*, 3–19.
17. Phan, R.; Seifman, M.A.; Dhillon, R.; Lim, P.; Hunter-Smith, D.J.; Rozen, W.M. Use of submental and submandibular free vascularized lymph node transfer for treatment of scrotal lymphedema: Report of two cases. *Microsurgery* **2020**, *40*, 808–813. [CrossRef] [PubMed]
18. Mikhael, M.; Khan, Y.S. Anatomy, Abdomen and Pelvis, Lymphatic Drainage. In *StatPearls*; StatPearls Publishing LLC.: Treasure Island, FL, USA, 2022.
19. Moellhoff, N.; Gernert, C.; Frank, K.; Giunta, R.E.; Ehrl, D. The 72-Hour Microcirculation Dynamics in Viable Free Flap Reconstructions. *J. Reconstr. Microsurg.* **2022**, *38*, 637–646. [CrossRef]
20. Szuba, A.; Shin, W.S.; Strauss, H.W.; Rockson, S. The third circulation: Radionuclide lymphoscintigraphy in the evaluation of lymphedema. *J. Nucl. Med.* **2003**, *44*, 43–57.
21. Schaverien, M.V.; Coroneos, C.J. Surgical Treatment of Lymphedema. *Plast. Reconstr. Surg.* **2019**, *144*, 738–758. [CrossRef]
22. Scaglioni, M.F.; Fontein, D.B.Y.; Arvanitakis, M.; Giovanoli, P. Systematic review of lymphovenous anastomosis (LVA) for the treatment of lymphedema. *Microsurgery* **2017**, *37*, 947–953. [CrossRef]
23. Ciudad, P.; Bolletta, A.; Kaciulyte, J.; Losco, L.; Manrique, O.J.; Cigna, E.; Mayer, H.F.; Escandón, J.M. The breast cancer-related lymphedema multidisciplinary approach: Algorithm for conservative and multimodal surgical treatment. *Microsurgery* **2023**, *43*, 427–436. [CrossRef] [PubMed]
24. Losco, L.; Bolletta, A.; de Sire, A.; Chen, S.H.; Sert, G.; Aksoyler, D.; Velazquez-Mujica, J.; Invernizzi, M.; Cigna, E.; Chen, H.C. The Combination of Lymph Node Transfer and Excisional Procedures in Bilateral Lower Extremity Lymphedema: Clinical Outcomes and Quality of Life Assessment with Long-Term Follow-Up. *J. Clin. Med.* **2022**, *11*, 570. [CrossRef] [PubMed]
25. Agko, M.; Ciudad, P.; Chen, H.C. Staged surgical treatment of extremity lymphedema with dual gastroepiploic vascularized lymph node transfers followed by suction-assisted lipectomy-A prospective study. *J. Surg. Oncol.* **2018**, *117*, 1148–1156. [CrossRef] [PubMed]

Disclaimer/Publisher's Note: The statements, opinions and data contained in all publications are solely those of the individual author(s) and contributor(s) and not of MDPI and/or the editor(s). MDPI and/or the editor(s) disclaim responsibility for any injury to people or property resulting from any ideas, methods, instructions or products referred to in the content.

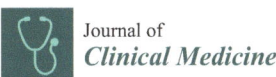

Article

Optimizing Orthognathic Surgery: Leveraging the Average Skull as a Dynamic Template for Surgical Simulation and Planning in 30 Patient Cases

Hsiu-Hsia Lin [1], Jyun-Cheng Kuo [2], Lun-Jou Lo [3] and Cheng-Ting Ho [4,*]

1. Craniofacial Research Center, Chang Gung Memorial Hospital, Taoyuan City 333, Taiwan; sharley@hust.edu.tw
2. Dental Department of TuCheng Hospital, New Taipei Municipal, New Taipei City 236, Taiwan; popop5541@cgmh.org.tw
3. Department of Plastic and Reconstructive Surgery, Craniofacial Research Center, Chang Gung Memorial Hospital, Chang Gung University, Taoyuan City 333, Taiwan; lunjoulo@cgmh.org.tw
4. Division of Craniofacial Orthodontics, Department of Dentistry, Chang Gung Memorial Hospital, Taoyuan City 333, Taiwan
* Correspondence: ma2589@gmail.com; Tel.: +886-3-328-1200 (ext. 2430); Fax: +886-3-327-1029

Abstract: Virtual planning has revolutionized orthognathic surgery (OGS), marking a significant advancement in the field. This study aims to showcase the practical application of our established 3D average skull template as a guiding framework for surgical planning, and to share valuable insights from our clinical experience. We enrolled 30 consecutive Taiwanese patients (18 females and 12 males) who underwent two-jaw orthognathic surgery with surgical simulation, utilizing the average skull template for planning. Results indicate the method's applicability and precision. By adhering to the surgical plan, post-operative outcomes closely aligned with the average skull template, showing negligible deviations of less than 2 mm. Moreover, patients expressed high satisfaction with post-surgery facial changes, with the chin appearance receiving the highest satisfaction scores, while the lowest scores were attributed to nose appearance. Notably, the substantial change in lower jaw position post-mandibular setback surgery contributed to increased satisfaction with the chin position. In conclusion, this study does not seek to replace established surgical planning methods, but underscores that utilizing an average skull as a surgical design template provides a viable, accurate, and efficient option for OGS patients.

Keywords: virtual planning; orthognathic surgery (OGS); average skull template; guiding framework; surgical simulation

1. Introduction

The evolution of digital technology and software has led to innovative approaches in orthognathic surgical (OGS) planning, enhancing its precision and efficiency. Traditional two-dimensional (2D) methods involving paper-based procedures and manual crafting have shifted to 3D technology applications, which overcome the limitations of time-consuming 2D methods and enhance detection in radiographs [1]. In the 3D field, simulations with dental casts using cone beam computed tomography (CBCT) and dental impression alternatives like oral scanning have emerged [2–5]. Despite the popularity of 3D methods, reliance on cephalometric measurements and norm values persists. A recent approach utilizing a three-dimensional average skull template for planning has been validated and applied in our center [6], streamlining the diagnosis of abnormal jaw positions and enabling surgery simulation without model surgery or angular measurements.

Class III malocclusion is prevalent in Asia (3–5% in Japan, around 2% in China) [7], where patients exhibit mandible prognathism, with or without maxillary retrognathism, which impacts their appearance and psychosocial status. Orthognathic surgery (OGS)

aims for a balanced facial profile, correct lower jaw positioning, and optimal dental occlusion [8,9]. Our prior research established a 3D cranial model integrated into virtual surgical planning (VSP) for repositioning the maxilla and mandible. For class III patients, OGS seeks to standardize jaw size, position, and aesthetics, which often involves mandibular setback using bilateral sagittal split osteotomy (BSSO) and maxillary advancement through LeFort I osteotomy. However, BSSO poses challenges, including potential inferior alveolar nerve injury.

Our previous study [6] demonstrated discrepancies of less than 1 mm in facial landmarks compared to 3D cephalometric measurements and surgical simulation with a 3D average skull template, validating its accuracy and clinical suitability.

This study aims to apply the average skull template to prospective patients, in order to guide surgical planning and evaluate outcomes and patient satisfaction for clinical dissemination. Future integration of artificial intelligence into surgical planning using the average skull template holds clinical potential [10–12]. Refined surgical planning simulations based on the average skull template and validated results will contribute to a machine learning facial classification model. The model will predict surgical plans for upcoming patients, providing initial references for clinical physicians, significantly reducing planning time and enhancing precision based on individual patient conditions and surgical assessments.

2. Materials and Methods

This study included 30 Taiwanese patients (18 females, 12 males) undergoing two-jaw orthognathic surgery (OGS) with surgical simulation using the average skull template, from August 2021 to July 2022. The patients, aged 22 to 38 years, presented with class III malocclusion, facial asymmetry, concave profile, and other related issues. All of them underwent cone beam computed tomography (CBCT) scans for surgical simulation. The procedures were performed by the same orthodontist and surgeon. Exclusions comprised severe deformities, prior orthognathic surgery, and facial trauma. Institutional Review Board approval was obtained (Chang Gung Medical Foundation IRB 202002305B0), and the participants provided informed consent. The methodology for constructing the 3D craniofacial model and 3D average skull-based surgical planning was outlined in a previous publication [6]. The study's flowchart (Figure 1) details four stages: 3D image acquisition, surgical simulation, actual surgery, and post-operative outcome validation.

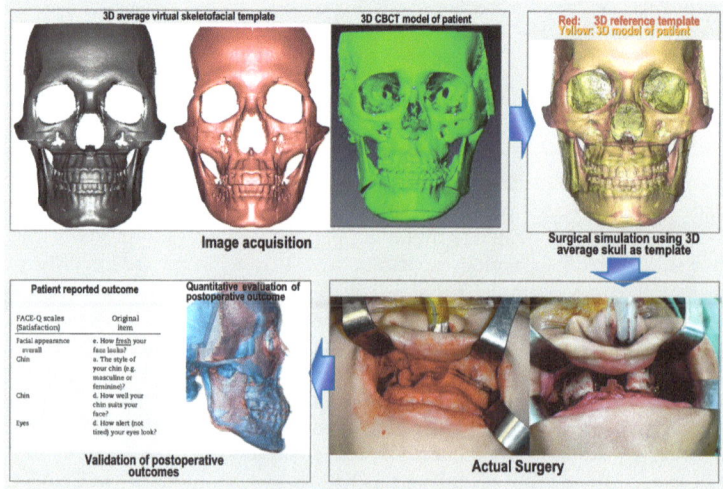

Figure 1. Flowchart of this prospective study's design.

2.1. Three-Dimensional Image Acquisition

Participants underwent pre-surgical CBCT scans using the KaVo ORTHOPANTOMO-GRAPH™ OP 3D Vision X-ray system (DEXIS™, Quakertown, PA, USA) with a low-dose protocol. The scans, performed 2 weeks pre-surgery, used 120 kVp, a voxel size of 0.4 mm × 0.4 mm × 0.4 mm, 26-s scan time, and an 11 cm × 23 cm × 17.3 cm field of view. Head orientation ensured that the Frankfort horizontal plane was parallel to the ground. The patients were instructed to avoid swallowing, to keep their mouths closed, and maintain a centric occlusion bite. The resulting DICOM-format image data, with 0.4 mm slice thickness, were processed in Materialise ProPlan CMF 3.0 (Leuven, Belgium) to reconstruct and analyze 3D bone and soft tissue models (Figure 2). Threshold values of 300–400 HU and 800–900 HU distinguished the hard and soft tissues, respectively. All CBCT data were stored in the Chang Gung Craniofacial Research Center's database.

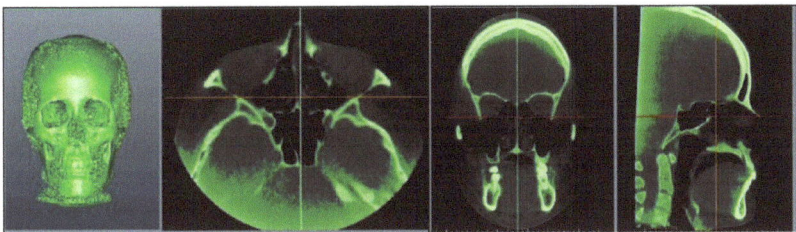

Figure 2. Reconstructing the 3D bone structure by importing 3D CBCT images.

2.2. Surgical Simulation Using 3D Average Skull as Template

The average skull served as a guide for surgical simulation, assessing deviations between two skull images in millimeters (sagittal, frontal, vertical). Using segmentation, the maxilla and mandible were delineated, and 3D CBCT dental structures were replaced with intra-oral scanner-acquired digital dental images using 3Shape, TRIOS® 3 (3Shape company, Copenhagen, Denmark). Dolphin Imaging® 11.95 software (Chatsworth, CA, United States) on the composite skull model established the virtual surgical occlusion setup, adjusting mandible position for normal overjet, overbite, midline alignment, and arch coordination. The setup considered a 15% surgical relapse with planned overcorrection (3–4 mm incisal overjet) in class III cases. Once the final virtual occlusion was confirmed, the maxilla and mandible were occluded to create the maxillomandibular complex object (MMC). Surgical simulation positioned the MMC close to the average skull template's maxillary, mandibular, and upper incisal positions (Figure 3) [6]. The three-step simulation process involves importing the 3D model template, identifying landmarks, superimposing the template and patient images, and conducting the simulation based on the MMC's position and pitch rotation. Detailed procedural descriptions are available in our previous publication [6].

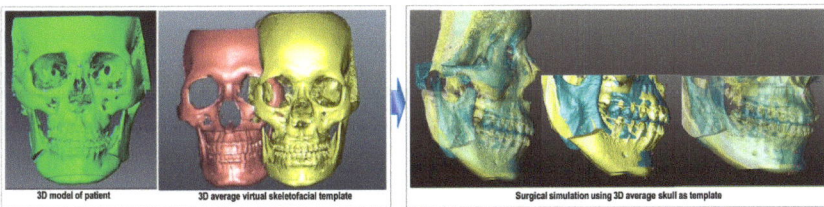

Figure 3. The surgical simulation using 3D average skull as template.

To validate the intra-observer reproducibility of landmark identification, 10 subjects were randomly selected for repeated testing. The defined landmarks were re-located in a

2-week interval by the same investigator (CT Ho). The intra-rater errors were analyzed by calculating the Euclidean distance between first and second landmarks' coordinates, A1 (X_{A1}, Y_{A1}, Z_{A1}) and A2 (X_{A2}, Y_{A2}, Z_{A2}), respectively, in a 3D coordinate system using the following formula:

$$\text{Distance}(d) = \sqrt{\left[(X_{A1} - X_{A2})^2 + (Y_{A1} - Y_{A2})^2 + (Z_{A1} - ZY_{A2})^2\right]}$$

2.3. Actual Surgery

We utilized a modified Hunsuck bilateral sagittal split osteotomy, LeFort I osteotomy, and, when necessary, genioplasty for all patients, following the single-splint two-jaw orthognathic surgery (OGS) method [13]. Full mobilization of the maxilla and mandible was achieved, adjusting the distal mandibular segment using the final occlusal splint to establish occlusion with the maxilla, creating the maxillomandibular complex (MMC). The MMC was repositioned based on the planned position, guided by a 3D average skull template through a customized positioning guide. Two guides were crafted using computer-aided design and manufacturing: one for LeFort I osteotomy, and another for positioning the MMC. The LeFort I guide was precisely placed on the maxilla to guide the osteotomy lines. After LeFort I osteotomy, the segments were secured onto the final occlusal splint. Using the positioning guide, the MMC was accurately relocated, temporarily secured with screws, and the facial skin was redraped for assessment. Lateral maxilla plate fixation followed, aligning the dental midline, skeletal midline, facial skin midline, occlusal plane, upper tooth show, facial proportion, and symmetry. The mandibular ramus fixation utilized percutaneous bicortical screws, with genioplasty if needed. Notably, guides were not used for mandibular ramus osteotomy, fixation, or genioplasty [14].

2.4. Validation of Post-Operative Outcomes

2.4.1. Quantitative Evaluation of Post-Operative Outcome

To assess the discrepancy between post-operative results and the average skull, 3D models were converted into stereolithography (STL) files for registration purposes. The average skull models were superimposed on the patients' skull models in the registration region (orbitale, frontal, the upper third or half of the nose, and external zygoma) based on seven pairs of anatomical landmarks (N, Or (L, R), Lo (L, R), Zy (L, R)), with image resizing performed to achieve the best alignment using the best-fit method in both the anterior and lateral views [14]. Subsequently, positional discrepancies (in millimeters) were evaluated at key anatomical points, including the maxilla (point A), the midcontact point of the upper incisors (U1C), the mandible (point B), and the chin (points Pog and Me). These image discrepancies pertaining to the maxilla, mandible, chin, and upper incisors were visualized and quantified using 3D software (Materialise ProPlan CMF 3.0), utilizing five pairs of anatomical landmarks (A, B, Pog, Me, U1).

2.4.2. Patient-Reported Outcome Questionnaires

Patients completed self-administered questionnaires to evaluate their facial appearance satisfaction six months post-surgery. This timing allowed for reduced facial swelling and enhanced tissue stability. Two measures were employed: overall appearance rating (OAR) and satisfaction with facial appearance (SFA) [14]. The OAR assesses ideal facial appearance perception on a 0 to 100 scale, with 1 being extremely unattractive and 10 extremely attractive. The SFA gauges satisfaction with specific features (nose, cheeks, lips, gum display, teeth, chin, and facial width) on a 1 to 10 scale, where 1 is very dissatisfied and 10 is very satisfied. Higher scores indicate increased satisfaction and facial attractiveness.

2.5. Statistical Analysis

The Pearson correlation coefficient was adopted to validate the intra-observer reproducibility. The range is between 0 and 1, with a higher value indicating a higher correlation or reliability. The means and standard deviations of the measurements were obtained for descriptive statistics. The data were verified to be normally distributed using the Kolmogorov–Smirnov test. The paired t-test was adopted for statistical comparisons between pre- and post-operative changes on cephalometric analysis. A p value of 0.05 was considered statistically significant. Statistical analyses were performed using SPSS Statistics for Windows, Version 17.0 (released 2008, SPSS Inc., Chicago, IL, USA).

3. Results

The mean intra-observer difference in landmark identification was 0.37 mm (range: 0.31–0.49 mm), and the Pearson correlation coefficients (r = 0.88–0.98; all $p < 0.05$) revealed significant correlations between the investigators' observations, indicating that the virtual-guided data collection was accurately and consistently performed (Table 1).

Table 1. Intra-observer reproducibility of landmark identification in the 3D coordinate system.

Landmark Definition	Mean Difference (mm)	r	p-Value
Nasion (N)	0.33	0.96	0.008 *
Lateral orbitale (Lo)	0.31	0.98	0.003 *
External Zygoma (Zy)	0.44	0.88	0.002 *
Orbitale (Or)	0.41	0.94	0.002 *
Anterior nasal spine (ANS)	0.40	0.91	0.006 *
A point (A)	0.34	0.93	0.008 *
B point (B)	0.35	0.89	0.005 *
Pogonion (Pog)	0.37	0.93	0.006 *
Menton (Me)	0.41	0.88	0.006 *
Gonion (Go)	0.49	0.88	0.006 *
U1 incisal tip (U1T)	0.31	0.99	0.003 *
U6 cusp (UR6C, UL6C)	0.37	0.98	0.006 *
L1 incisal tip (L1T)	0.34	0.93	0.005 *
L6 cusp (LR6C LL6C)	0.42	0.92	0.003 *
Mean ± SD	0.37 ± 0.067		

r, Pearson correlation coefficient; * $p < 0.05$.

Table 2 presents the differences between post-operative results and the average skull. The mean differences were computed in three anatomical planes: the transverse plane (x-axis, mediolateral), the sagittal plane (y-axis, anteroposterior), and the vertical plane (z-axis, superiorinferior). The study did not include patients with positional differences exceeding 3 mm in any direction. All of the data points exhibited deviations of less than 2 mm, except for Pog in the anteroposterior direction (2.3 mm). U1 mid in the y-axis displayed a measurement discrepancy of 1.9 mm, and Me in the vertical direction showed a deviation of 1.9 mm, which closely approached the 2 mm threshold. This suggests a tendency toward greater alignment in the x-axis for all landmarks compared to the y- and z-axes, as measurements in the x-axis were smaller than those in the other two axes. Furthermore, there was less deviation observed in the maxilla (point A) than in the mandible (points B and Pog) in all three axes. Notably, the maxilla (A point, x = 0.9, y = 1.1, z = 1.0) exhibited the highest degree of alignment among all landmarks. This study introduces a novel approach, and as of now, substantial results are not directly available. Following the "rule of thumb" established in previous studies, we conducted initial testing with a sample size of 30 [15]. A sample size of 30 is sufficient for a post hoc power analysis of 0.75 to detect the difference.

Table 2. Differences between images obtained using 3D cephalometric normative data and average 3D skeletofacial model for male participants.

Parameters	Mediolateral	Anteroposterior	Superoinferior	p-Value
A point	0.975 ± 0.805	1.150 ± 1.008	1.088 ± 0.686	0.885
U1 mid	1.066 ± 0.704	1.940 ± 2.082	1.216 ± 0.883	0.172
B point	1.379 ± 1.259	1.205 ± 0.570	1.276 ± 0.832	0.908
Pog	1.475 ± 1.338	2.357 ± 0.930	1.395 ± 1.397	0.148
Me	1.627 ± 1.376	1.672 ± 1.285	1.925 ± 1.341	0.854

Data are in millimeters and are presented as mean ± standard deviation. A sample size of 30 is sufficient for a post hoc power analysis of 0.75 to detect the difference.

The overall appearance rating (OAR) and satisfaction with facial appearance (SFA) results are shown in Table 3. The highest level of satisfaction was observed in terms of chin appearance, while the lowest score was recorded for nose appearance. All of the scores were close to 9, indicating a high level of satisfaction. A significant alteration in the position of the lower jaw following mandibular setback may contribute to a higher satisfaction score for chin position.

Table 3. The overall appearance rating (OAR) and satisfaction with facial appearance of patient-reported outcomes.

Scale	Orthognathic Surgery-Treated Patients		
	Total	Male	Female
	(n = 30)	(n = 18)	(n = 12)
Overall appearance rating (0–100)	89.6 ± 7.6	88.3 ± 8.7	89.8 ± 7.2
Facial area satisfaction (0–10)			
Cheek fullness	8.7 ± 0.9	8.8 ± 1.0	8.5 ± 0.7
Chin	9.1 ± 0.9	9.1 ± 1.0	9.1 ± 0.9
Nose	8.3 ± 1.1 *	8.4 ± 1.1 *	8.2 ± 1.2
Lip	8.9 ± 1.1	8.6 ± 1.3	9.3 ± 0.4
Gum show	8.9 ± 0.9	8.9 ± 1.1	8.9 ± 0.7
Dental alignment	9.0 ± 0.9	8.9 ± 0.9	9.2 ± 0.8
facial width change	8.6 ± 0.8	8.5 ± 0.6	8.6 ± 0.8

Data presented as mean ± standard deviation. Higher scores indicate higher satisfaction. * represents the item with the lowest satisfaction.

4. Discussion

Leveraging 3D simulation techniques provides a distinct advantage in refining surgical planning precision by adjusting the yaw, roll, and pitch rotation of the osteotomized bony segment. Additionally, the 3D simulation detects and addresses collisions or gaps between bony segments, leading to improved surgical outcomes. Moreover, it expedites treatment planning and proves to be a more cost-effective alternative compared to traditional methods [16–18].

To our knowledge, this marks the first assessment of treatment outcomes in patients with class III malocclusion and facial asymmetry undergoing two-jaw surgery, utilizing a 3D average skull as a reference template for surgical planning. The study has limitations in terms of its generalizability, as the sample for the average skull template comprises only normal subjects from Taiwan, making it primarily applicable to Chinese or Asian populations. However, the methodology can be extended to address malocclusions or facial deformities more broadly. Another limitation is the static approach of the study, as it focused on hard tissue surgical simulation using an average template, which makes it challenging to accurately predict soft tissue changes and dynamics, such as gum exposure during smiling. Videos could serve as a valuable tool for dynamically assessing and recording soft tissue, necessitating a final adjustment to the surgical plan after clinical evaluation. Therefore, final modifications are still needed after clinical evaluation for dynamic soft tissue expression.

Accurately predicting post-operative facial appearance during surgical planning simulation requires a comprehensive understanding of the relationship between the displacement of soft tissues and bone tissues (hard tissues) before and after surgery. This understanding, which is not limited to specific regions, necessitates a holistic approach (non-localized analysis) that acknowledges that the proportion is not one-to-one. To address this, we plan to utilize deep learning techniques to establish a three-dimensional orthognathic surgery soft tissue prediction simulation system. Facial regions impacted by surgery will be subdivided into smaller areas, each with its pre- and post-operative skeletal displacement values (input) and soft tissue displacement values (output). We aim to leverage artificial intelligence (AI) technology, specifically convolutional neural network (CNN), to build a facial soft tissue prediction model. Clinically, this approach enables physicians not only to adjust surgical plans (skeletal displacement) based on predicted facial outcomes, but also to provide a realistic preview of post-surgery facial appearance, acting as a communication tool for easy patient understanding.

Using an average skull as a surgical design model does not aim to replace the current method, but provides a valuable alternative. Compared to existing surgical simulation protocols, our method stands out. Unlike other approaches that require 3D cephalometric analysis involving angular and linear measurements and reliance on norm values to plan osteotomized bony segments, our study is significantly more efficient. We eliminate the need for cephalometric analysis and dental models. By superimposing two skull images, we visualize and calculate deviations from the ideal position in linear measurements across three coordinates. This streamlines the process and enhances communication and education with patients. However, it is important to note that our approach is static, focusing on the average skull model without considering the dynamics of soft tissues.

In our investigation, we utilized Dolphin imaging 11.95 to integrate intra-oral scans with CBCT scans for dental fusion. The accuracy of this fusion process, assessed using commercially available software, demonstrated a high level of precision compared to the established gold standard. Although there may be some inaccuracies in the cranial/caudal directions for both the maxilla and mandible, we addressed this by employing fiducial markers and the best-fit method to refine the fusion process [19]. Nonetheless, a visual check is recommended. To further enhance accuracy in aligning intra-oral scans with dental surfaces in CBCT, we employed fiducial markers and the best-fit method in fusing dental elements from intra-oral scans. Again, a visual check is advised for validation [20].

In this study, we compared positional disparities between the post-operative skull and the average skull using paired landmarks, and administered patient satisfaction questionnaires concerning overall appearance and specific facial regions. These questionnaires, which are validated instruments for patients following orthognathic surgery, assessed perception of appearance with two measures: overall appearance rating (OAR) and satisfaction with facial appearance (SFA) [14]. Minimal jaw bone deviations were observed between paired landmarks, and the patient-reported satisfaction levels were notably high. The success of orthognathic surgery relies on precise surgical planning and patient contentment. This innovative approach presents an alternative tool for virtual 3D surgical planning of orthognathic surgery.

Based on the results in Table 2, three-dimensional analysis revealed minimal discrepancies between the post-operative skull and the average skull template for specific paired landmarks, including point A (maxilla), U1, point B (mandible), Pog, and Me. Most of these paired landmark deviations were small, measuring less than 2 mm in absolute value, except for Pog, which exhibited a 2.3 mm deviation in the anteroposterior direction. Previous studies recommended a 2 mm range as the most suitable criterion for assessing linear differences between planned and actual post-operative images [21–23]. Our results fell within this recommended range. The slight anterior shift of Pog by 0.3 mm beyond this range could be attributed to mild relapse in the lower jaw six months post-surgery, influenced by muscular actions on bony tissue, condylar changes, or other contributing factors [24]. The second-largest deviation was observed in the vertical difference at Me (1.9 mm, still less than 2 mm), possibly explained by the facial patterns of selected patients. The facial index range for mesocephalic patterns typically falls within 0.85–0.89 (N-Me/Zy-Zy). Some patients with longer or shorter faces within this range may influence the average data, but the deviations still fall within the 2 mm margin criteria. Regarding U1 mid, exhibiting a 1.9 mm deviation in the y-axis, this can be attributed to the modified surgical approach in our protocol. Minimal dental decompensation was performed before surgery, and any remaining discrepancies can be readily corrected through post-surgical orthodontic treatment. Hsu et al. demonstrated that the precision of surgical simulation in orthognathic surgery can result in deviations ranging from 0.6 to 3.5 mm from the virtual plan [25]. Therefore, our study, utilizing this novel method, can aid in presurgical planning and maintain accuracy in orthognathic surgery.

This study demonstrates a higher level of congruence when comparing the deviation of the actual post-operative results to the average skull template in the maxilla (point A, $x = 0.9$ mm, $y = 1.1$ mm, $z = 1.0$ mm) compared to the mandible (point B, $x = 1.3$ mm, $y = 1.2$ mm, $z = 1.2$ mm, and Me, $x = 1.6$ mm, $y = 1.6$ mm, $z = 1.9$ mm) in three-dimensional space. It can be hypothesized that the mandible is occluded with the maxilla, and the chin is distant from the rotation center (maxilla), resulting in less conformity in the lower jaw position due to the longer radius effect from the rotation center. In other words, a smaller deviation in the maxilla may lead to a larger deviation in the mandible. In this study, the highest degree of conformity was observed in the mediolateral direction in all landmarks compared to the y- and z-axes, consistent with our previous reports, where more favorable outcomes were noted in frontal symmetry (x-axis, mediolateral direction) in midsagittal plane landmarks when comparing the 3D planning group to the 2D planning group. This finding aligns with the report by Alex Wilson et al. [23]. However, our study observed clinically insignificant deviations in the vertical height of the maxilla (A point 1.0 mm in the z-axis). This result contradicts the findings of Alex Wilson et al., who reported the greatest nonconformity in the vertical plane (points A and B). We speculate that the routine use of a positional guide to guide the maxilla into the planned position during surgery in our center may contribute to less error in locating the maxilla [14]. In contrast, Alex et al. used vertical measurements from an external reference point, using the medial canthus to fixed dental landmarks without a bone-to-bone guide, which could result in larger deviations in the vertical direction. We observed an incongruence in the sagittal positioning of the chin (Pog), consistent with Alex Wilson et al., and this discrepancy could be attributed to changes in condylar position or relapse.

To address patient preferences and evaluate post-surgery satisfaction, we administered a patient-reported outcome questionnaire [25–27]. According to Table 3, patients exhibited high satisfaction with their overall appearance (scores near 90) when utilizing the average skull template for surgical planning. This heightened satisfaction may positively impact their self-confidence and social interactions. Concerning specific facial areas, the nose received the lowest score (8.3). Some patients expressed worries about nostril base enlargement or a flattened nasal bridge following Le Fort I osteotomy. Changes of this nature could be attributed to the detachment of subnasal soft tissues and muscles during the osteotomy. Main V et al. reported a mean increase in alar base width of 1.176 mm in Le Fort I osteotomy patients [28]. Trevisiol et al. demonstrated an increase in inter-alar width of 1.7 mm in patients who underwent subspinal Le Fort I osteotomy [29]. Mitigating strategies, such as an alar base cinch suture or rhinoplasty, may help address these undesirable nasal aesthetic changes [30]. Some patients expressed dissatisfaction with a broader facial appearance in the frontal view following BSSO setback (score 8.6). This phenomenon is thought to result from an increase in intergonial width and bone overlap in the proximal and distal segments during mandibular setback [31–34]. Yoshioka et al. reported a 0.45 mm increase in intergonial width in the SSRO group [33]. Choi et al. reported a 2.1 mm increase in intergonial width after SSRO [34]. Chen et al. noted a nonsignificant increase of 1.2 mm in intergonial widths with SSRO setback [32]. However, this phenomenon appeared to normalize and become insignificant over time through bone remodeling [34].

In comparison to Hsu's study on the accuracy of the CASS protocol for orthognathic surgery, our results showed similarities in the range of positional differences between virtual plans and actual results (0.97–2.35 mm vs. 0.6–3.5 mm), meeting the accepted clinical threshold of 2 mm. However, their method involves collecting anthropometric measurements, stone models, and a patient-specific bite jig, facebow, orientation sensor, and CT scan before surgical simulation, which makes this approach more time-consuming and complex. In our study, we used intra-oral scans to obtain digital dental images for fusing dentition from intra-oral scans in CBCT scans. When the patient's skull was superimposed on the 3D average template, deviations could easily be visualized and calculated without the need for extensive anthropometric measurements and stone models. Comparing the overall appearance scores in this study to our previous study, which used 3D cephalometric norms as a guideline for surgical planning, both methods yielded similar satisfaction scores (89.6 ± 7.6 vs. 89.7 ± 4.5). Furthermore, these scores surpassed those reported by Liao et al. (89.6 ± 7.6 vs. 82.0 ± 11.8) in their study, where they employed a surgical-first approach for orthognathic surgery [18]. This suggests that our new method is as effective as the currently established approach, but offers the advantages of simplicity, time efficiency, and enhanced surgical planning effectiveness.

While the average skull template proves to be a valuable tool, the ultimate decision still relies on soft tissue considerations, such as ex paranasal depression, incisor exposure, and soft tissue chin thickness, as the 3D template method is static rather than dynamic. Experienced doctors may discern potential surgical plans upon initial clinical evaluation. However, with the aid of this template, they can easily validate their diagnoses, particularly in borderline cases. For less experienced practitioners, this template can serve as a starting point for learning how to accurately diagnose maxillary retrusion, mandibular prognathism, or a combination of both in class III malocclusion cases. Therefore, it proves to be a valuable tool for both training purposes and clinical application.

There has been an evolution in virtual planning for orthognathic surgery (OGS), transitioning from 2D methods to 3D methods, with potential future applications involving artificial intelligence (AI). Our previous preliminary study, which utilized an average 3D skull template as a reference for surgical planning to reposition the maxilla and mandible, demonstrated a high level of consistency with simulation images generated using 3D cephalometric normative data, particularly in terms of jawbone positioning [6]. We believe that long-term follow-up (2–3 years later) would better evaluate its stability for OGS. In our study, we propose a new method of surgical simulation, and the planned jaw bone position using our method is similar to other VSP (virtual surgical planning). However, overcorrection is needed to compensate for possible surgical relapse in severe class III malocclusion. The objective of this study is to assess post-operative outcomes and patient satisfaction with this novel surgical planning method, recognizing that patient-reported outcomes hold great value in evaluating the practicality of new techniques. The results indicate that all post-operative data closely align with the average skull template, and patients express high levels of satisfaction, underscoring the reliability of this method for surgical planning. This approach is straightforward and efficient for diagnosis and the establishment of surgical plans.

5. Conclusions

This research offers a precise and efficient alternative for OGS patients, aiding communication with patients and educating young doctors. Future possibilities include integrating AI technology to generate diagnoses and surgical plans swiftly by inputting a patient's 3D image into the software.

Author Contributions: Conception and design: C.-T.H. and H.-H.L.; acquisition, analysis, and interpretation of data: C.-T.H. and J.-C.K.; drafting of the article: C.-T.H. and H.-H.L.; critical revision of the article: C.-T.H. and L.-J.L.; study supervision: C.-T.H.; review of the submitted version of the manuscript: all authors. All authors have read and agreed to the published version of the manuscript.

Funding: This research was funded by a grant from Chang Gung Memorial Hospital (CMRPG3L1711).

Institutional Review Board Statement: This study was performed with the approval of the Institutional Review Board (Chang Gung Medical Foundation IRB 202002305B0).

Informed Consent Statement: Informed consent was obtained from all subjects involved in the study.

Data Availability Statement: The data presented in this study is available upon request to the corresponding author. As the data belongs to the hospital, it is not publicly accessible.

Acknowledgments: The authors would like to express their appreciation to Min-Chi Chen from the Department of Public Health and Biostatistics Consulting Center, School of Medicine, Chang Gung University, for conducting the statistical analysis.

Conflicts of Interest: The authors declare no conflict of interest with respect to the authorship or publication of this article.

References

1. Narayan, H.G.; ChaiKiat, C. Orthodontic-orthognathic interventions in orthognathic surgical cases: "Paper surgery" and "model surgery" concepts in surgical orthodontics. *Contemp. Clin. Dent.* **2016**, *7*, 386–390.
2. Xia, J.J.; Gateno, J.; Teichgraeber, J.F. New clinical protocol to evaluate craniomaxillofacial deformity and plan surgical correction. *J. Oral. Maxillofac. Surg.* **2009**, *67*, 2093–2106. [CrossRef] [PubMed]
3. Naidu, D.; Freer, T.J. Validity, reliability, and reproducibility of the iOC intraoral scanner: A comparison of tooth widths and Bolton ratios. *Am. J. Orthod. Dentofacial Orthop.* **2013**, *144*, 304–310. [CrossRef] [PubMed]
4. Zimmermann, M.; Mehl, A.M.; Mörmann, W.H.; Reich, S. Intraoral scanning systems: A current overview. *Int. J. Comput. Dent.* **2015**, *18*, 101–129. [PubMed]
5. Grünheid, T.; McCarthy, S.D.; Larson, B.E. Clinical use of a direct chairside oral scanner: An assessment of accuracy, time, and patient acceptance. *Am. J. Orthod. Dentofacial Orthop.* **2014**, *146*, 673–682. [CrossRef] [PubMed]
6. Ho, C.T.; Denadai, R.; Lo, L.J.; Lin, H.H. Average 3D Skeletofacial Model as a Template for Maxillomandibular Repositioning During Virtual Orthognathic Surgical Planning. *Plast. Reconstr. Surg.* **2023**, *21*, 10–97. [CrossRef] [PubMed]
7. Proffit, W.R.; Fields, H.W.; Larson, B.; Sarver, D.M. *Contemporary Orthodontics*, 6th ed.; Mosby Inc.: Maryland Heights, MO, USA, 2013.
8. Bayome, M.; Park, J.H.; Kook, Y.A. New three-dimensional cephalometric analyses among adults with a skeletal class I pattern and normal occlusion. *Korean J. Orthod.* **2013**, *43*, 62–73. [CrossRef] [PubMed]
9. Cheung, L.K.; Chan, Y.M.; Jayaratne, Y.S.; Lo, J. Three-dimensional cephalometric norms of Chinese adults in Hong Kong with balanced facial profile. *Oral. Surg. Oral. Med. Oral. Pathol. Oral. Radiol. Endod.* **2011**, *112*, e56–e73. [CrossRef]
10. Lo, L.J.; Yang, C.T.; Ho, C.T.; Liao, C.H.; Lin, H.H. Automatic Assessment of 3-Dimensional Facial Soft Tissue Symmetry Before and After Orthognathic Surgery Using a Machine Learning Model: A Preliminary Experience. *Ann. Plast. Surg.* **2021**, *3S* (Suppl. S2), S224–S228. [CrossRef]
11. Zhou, X.Y.; Guo, Y.; Shen, M.; Yang, G.Z. Application of artificial intelligence in surgery. *Front. Med.* **2020**, *14*, 417–430. [CrossRef]
12. Bhandari, M.; Zeffiro, T.; Reddiboina, M. Artificial intelligence and robotic surgery: Current perspective and future directions. *Curr. Opin. Urol.* **2020**, *30*, 48–54. [CrossRef] [PubMed]
13. Bergeron, L.; Yu, C.C.; Chen, Y.R. Single-splint technique for correction of severe facial asymmetry: Correlation between intraoperative maxillomandibular complex roll and restoration of mouth symmetry. *Plast. Reconstr. Surg.* **2008**, *122*, 1535–1541. [CrossRef] [PubMed]
14. Lo, L.J.; Lin, H.H. Applications of three-dimensional imaging techniques in craniomaxillofacial surgery: A literature review. *Biomed. J.* **2023**, *46*, 100615. [CrossRef] [PubMed]
15. Browne, R.H. On the use of a pilot sample for sample size determination. *Stat. Med.* **1995**, *14*, 1933–1940. [CrossRef] [PubMed]
16. Steinhuber, T.; Brunold, S.; Gärtner, C.; Offermanns, V.; Ulmer, H.; Ploder, O. Is virtual surgical planning in orthognathic surgery faster than conventional planning? A time and workflow analysis of an office-based workflow for single-and double-jaw surgery. *J. Oral. Maxillofac. Surg.* **2018**, *76*, 397–407. [CrossRef] [PubMed]
17. Wrzosek, M.K.; Peacock, Z.S.; Laviv, A.; Goldwaser, B.R.; Ortiz, R.; Resnick, C.M.; Troulis, M.J.; Kaban, L.B. Comparison of time required for traditional versus virtual orthognathic surgery treatment planning. *Int. J. Oral. Maxillofac. Surg.* **2016**, *45*, 1065–1069. [CrossRef] [PubMed]
18. Donaldson, C.D.; Manisali, M.; Naini, F.B. Three-dimensional virtual surgical planning (3D-VSP) in orthognathic surgery: Advantages, disadvantages and pitfalls. *J. Orthod.* **2021**, *48*, 52–63. [CrossRef] [PubMed]
19. Lin, H.H.; Chiang, W.C.; Lo, L.J.; Hsu, S.P.; Wang, C.H.; Wan, S.Y. Artifact-resistant superimposition of digital dental models and cone-beam computed tomography images. *J. Oral. Maxillofac. Surg.* **2013**, *71*, 1933–1947. [CrossRef]

20. Baan, F.; Bruggink, R.; Nijsink, J.; Maal, T.J.J.; Ongkosuwito, E.M. Fusion of intra-oral scans in cone-beam computed tomography scans. *Clin. Oral. Investig.* **2021**, *25*, 77–85. [CrossRef]
21. Liao1, Y.F.; Chen, Y.F.; Yao, C.F.; Chen, Y.A.; Chen, Y.R. Long-term outcomes of bimaxillary surgery for treatment of asymmetric skeletal class III deformity using surgery-first approach. *Clin. Oral. Investig.* **2019**, *23*, 1685–1693. [CrossRef]
22. Holte, M.B.; Diaconu, A.; Ingerslev, J.; Thorn, J.J.; Pinholt, E.M. Virtual Analysis of Segmental Bimaxillary Surgery: A Validation Study. *J. Oral. Maxillofac. Surg.* **2021**, *79*, 2320–2333. [CrossRef]
23. Wilson, A.; Gabrick, K.; Wu, R.; Madari, S.; Sawh-Martinez, R.; Steinbacher, D. Conformity of the Actual to the Planned Result in Orthognathic Surgery. *Plast. Reconstr. Surg.* **2019**, *144*, 89e–97e. [CrossRef] [PubMed]
24. de Haan, I.F.; Ciesielski, R.; Nitsche, T.; Koos, B. Evaluation of relapse after orthodontic therapy combined with orthognathic surgery in the treatment of skeletal class III. *J. Orofac. Orthop.* **2013**, *74*, 362–369. [CrossRef] [PubMed]
25. Hsu, S.S.; Gateno, J.; Bell, R.B.; Hirsch, D.L.; Markiewicz, M.R.; Teichgraeber, J.F.; Zhou, X.; Xia, J.J. Accuracy of a computeraided surgical simulation protocol for orthognathic surgery: A prospective multicenter study. *J. Oral. Maxillofac. Surg.* **2013**, *71*, 128–142. [CrossRef] [PubMed]
26. Nelson, E.C.; Eftimovska, E.; Lind, C.; Hager, A.; Wasson, J.H.; Lindblad, S. Patient reported outcome measures in practice. *BMJ* **2015**, *350*, g7818. [CrossRef] [PubMed]
27. Lee, L.W.; Chen, S.H.; Yu, C.C.; Lo, L.J.; Lee, S.R.; Chen, Y.R. Stigma, body image, and quality of life in women seeking orthognathic surgery. *Plast. Reconstr. Surg.* **2007**, *120*, 225–231. [CrossRef] [PubMed]
28. Mani, V.; Panicker, P.; Shenoy, A.; George, A.L.; Chacko, T. Evaluation of Changes in the Alar Base Width Following Lefort 1 and AMO with Conventional Alar Cinch Suturing: A Photographic Study of 100 Cases. *J. Maxillofac. Oral. Surg.* **2020**, *19*, 21–25. [CrossRef]
29. Trevisiol, L.; Lanaro, L.; Favero, V.; Lonardi, F.; Vania, M.; D'Agostino, A. The effect of subspinal Le Fort I osteotomy and alar cinch suture on nasal widening. *J. Craniomaxillofac Surg.* **2020**, *48*, 832–838. [CrossRef]
30. Howley, C.; Ali, N.; Lee, R.; Cox, S. Use of the alar base cinch suture in Le Fort I osteotomy: Is it effective? *Br. J. Oral. Maxillofac. Surg.* **2011**, *49*, 127–130. [CrossRef]
31. Chen, C.M.; Tseng, Y.C.; Ko, E.C.; Chen, M.Y.C.; Chen, K.J.; Cheng, J.H. Comparisons of Jaw Line and Face Line after Mandibular Setback: Intraoral Vertical Ramus versus Sagittal Split Ramus Osteotomie. *Biomed. Res. Int.* **2018**, *2*, 1–7. [CrossRef]
32. Chen, C.M.; Chen Michael, Y.C.; Cheng, J.H.; Chen, K.J.; Tseng, Y.C. Facial profile and frontal changes after bimaxillary surgery in patients with mandibular prognathism. *J. Formos. Med. Assoc.* **2018**, *117*, 632–639. [CrossRef]
33. Yoshioka, I.; Khanal, A.; Tominaga, K.; Horie, A.; Furuta, N.; Fukuda, J. Vertical ramus versus sagittal split osteotomies: Comparison of stability after mandibular setback. *J. Oral. Maxillofac. Surg.* **2008**, *66*, 1138–1144. [CrossRef]
34. Choi, Y.J.; Ha, Y.D.; Lim, H.; Huh, J.K.; Chung, C.J.; Kim, K.H. Long-term changes in mandibular and facial widths afer mandibular setback surgery using intraoral vertical ramus osteotomy. *Int. J. Oral. Maxillofac. Surg.* **2016**, *45*, 1074–1080. [CrossRef]

Disclaimer/Publisher's Note: The statements, opinions and data contained in all publications are solely those of the individual author(s) and contributor(s) and not of MDPI and/or the editor(s). MDPI and/or the editor(s) disclaim responsibility for any injury to people or property resulting from any ideas, methods, instructions or products referred to in the content.

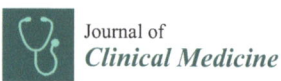
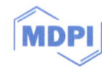

Article

How to Treat a Cyclist's Nodule?—Introduction of a Novel, ICG-Assisted Approach

Julius M. Mayer [1,*,†], Sophie I. Spies [2,†], Carla K. Mayer [3], Cédric Zubler [1], Rafael Loucas [4] and Thomas Holzbach [4]

[1] Department of Plastic and Hand Surgery, Inselspital, University Hospital Bern, 3010 Bern, Switzerland; cedric.zubler@insel.ch
[2] Department of Dermatology and Allergy, Technical University Munich, 80802 Munich, Germany
[3] Department of Urology, Spital Thurgau, 8500 Frauenfeld, Switzerland
[4] Department of Hand and Plastic Surgery, Spital Thurgau, 8500 Frauenfeld, Switzerland; rafael.loucas@stgag.ch (R.L.); thomas.holzbach@stgag.ch (T.H.)
* Correspondence: julius.m.mayer@gmail.com
† These authors contributed equally to this work.

Abstract: Background: Perineal nodular induration (PNI) is a benign proliferation of the soft tissue in the perineal region that is associated with saddle sports, especially road cycling. The etiology has not been conclusively clarified; however, repeated microtrauma to the collagen and subcutaneous fat tissue by pressure, vibration and shear forces is considered a mechanical pathomechanism. In this context, chronic lymphedema resulting in the development of fibrous tissue has been suggested as an etiological pathway of PNI. The primary aim of this study was to introduce and elucidate a novel operative technique regarding PNI that is assisted by indocyanine green (ICG). In order to provide some context for this approach, we conducted a comprehensive review of the existing literature. This dual objective aimed to contribute to the existing body of knowledge while introducing an innovative surgical approach for managing PNI. Methods: We reviewed publications relating to PNI published between 1990 and 2023. In addition to the thorough review of the literature, we presented our novel surgical approach. We described how this elaborate approach for extensive cases of PNI involves surgical excision combined with tissue doubling and intraoperative ICG visualization for exact lymphatic vessel obliteration to minimize the risk of recurrence based on the presumed context of lymphatic congestion. Results: The literature research yielded 16 PubMed articles encompassing 23 cases of perineal nodular induration (PNI) or cyclist's nodule. Of these, 9 cases involved females, and 14 involved males. Conservative treatment was documented in 7 cases (30%), while surgical approaches were reported in 16 cases (70%). Notably, a limited number of articles focused on histopathological or radiological characteristics, with a shortage of structured reviews on surgical treatment options. Only two articles provided detailed insights into surgical techniques. Similarly to the two cases of surgical intervention identified in the literature research, the post-operative recovery in our ICG assisted surgical approach was prompt, meaning a return to cycling was possible six weeks after surgery. At the end of the observation period (twelve months after surgery), regular scar formation and no signs of recurrence were seen. Conclusion: We hope that this article draws attention to the condition of PNI in times of increasing popularity of cycling as a sport. We aimed to contribute to the existing body of knowledge through our thorough review of the existing literature while introducing an innovative surgical approach for managing PNI. Due to the successful outcome, the combination of tissue doubling, intraoperative ICG visualization and postoperative negative wound therapy should be considered as a therapeutic strategy in cases of large PNI.

Keywords: cyclist's nodule; perineal nodular induration; perineal tumor; third testicle; impaired lymphatic drainage; indocyanine green; ICG; plastic surgery; epicutaneous negative wound therapy; road cycling

1. Introduction

Perineal nodular induration (PNI), more commonly known as "third testicle" or "cyclist's nodule" [1], is a rare and benign (myo)fibroblastic pseudotumor associated with saddle sports, such as cycling or horseback-riding [2–6]. The clinical appearance of PNI is characterized by unspecific swelling of the soft tissue posterior at the perineum or over the ischial tuberosity [7]. The PNI manifests as two nodules, with one on each side of the perineal raphe; in other cases, it presents as a single nodule [1]. This localization of the swelling led to reports in journals on various medical disciplines, such as urology [2,8], gynecology [9,10], dermatology [1,3], orthopedic surgery [11] and plastic surgery, as well as histopathology [4,12] and radiology [13–15]. Overall, PNI is a rare disease and the knowledge about its treatment is limited. Between 1990–2023, a total of 16 PubMed listed articles involving 23 cases were published on the search term "perineal nodular induration or cyclist's nodule". Of these, 9 cases concerned female patients and 14 cases male patients. In 7 of the 23 (30%) cases, conservative treatment was described, while in 16 of the 23 cases (70%), surgical treatment approaches were discussed. Some of the 16 articles focused more on histopathological or radiological characteristics than on treatment options. To our knowledge, a structured review article on surgical treatment options is not yet available. Only two of these articles gave further insight into detailed surgical techniques. In one article, a spindle-shaped mass excision and wound closure by bilateral advancement flaps was mentioned [2]. Respectively, an incision at the lateral side of the perineum and a resection of the mass and simple wound closure was described in the other [16].

Histologically, a PNI is most likely the result of repeated microtrauma to the collagen and subcutaneous fat tissue by pressure, shear forces and vibration. Microtrauma can cause fibrinoid collagen degeneration with myxoid changes, pseudocysts formation and potential lymphatic vessel impairment [1]. Formation of a lymphatic drainage disorder can occur and result in chronic non-healing wounds. Although the etiology of PNI is not conclusively established, similarities in the clinical appearance to lymphedema have been observed. There is evidence in terms of similar appearance, continuous development with continued exposure and fibrotic remodeling during progression. For example, the altered skin with, in some cases, non-healing sores in advanced conditions resembles that of advanced chronic lymphedema skin alterations. One may suspect a relationship between the condition and a pressure/shear force-related chronic lymphatic drainage problem, and, indeed, in some histopathological examinations, obliterated and fibrosed lymphatic vessels were seen [9,17].

To the best of our knowledge, a proper classification of PNI has not yet been established. In our opinion, based on the size of the mass (small/medium/large in proportion to the total perineal area and the height of the tumor) and the patient's discomfort, one might scale the PNI and decide on possible treatment options. For small lesions, conversative treatment is applicable. This includes the alteration of the cause, namely adjustment of the rider's position on the saddle and wearing appropriate cycling pants. Rest alone was reported as not resulting in spontaneous regression of the mass [2,15]. However, further progression could be stopped by avoiding cycling. Complex physical decongestive therapy (CDT) is rarely mentioned in the context of PNI. Nevertheless, if PNI is pathogenetically related to lymphatic congestion, then conservative treatment strategies for lymphedema should be also considered for mild findings of PNI. The standard therapy for lymphedema is CDT, which consists of the following coordinated components: skin care and, if necessary, skin rehabilitation and manual lymphatic drainage, supplemented with additive manual techniques, compression therapy, education and instruction on self-treatment [18]. In a few case reports of small to medium PNIs, intralesional corticosteroid or hyaluronidase injections were found to offer some relief; however, these injections may cause subcutaneous atrophy [3,16,19,20]. These techniques are insufficient or, in some cases, even contraindicated in the setting of late-stage lymphedema and/or extensive tissue fibrosis (as late-stage PNIs), necessitating a more radical approach in terms of surgical excision. We describe our surgical treatment of extensive late-stage PNIs with a previously unreported technique based on the presumed context of lymphatic congestion using intraoperative ICG-monitoring for exact lymphatic vessel obliteration, which should minimize recurrence risk and allow for a prompt return to cycling.

The clinical utilization of ICG has attained a well-established status in the field of plastic surgery. The ICG technique entails the intravenous or intradermal administration of a fluorescent solution, namely Verdye, in our hands (5 mg/mL, Diagnostic Green GmbH, München, Germany). This dye expeditiously forms complexes with plasma proteins and exhibits near-infrared fluorescence upon exposure to specific wavelengths. Within the realm of plastic surgery, surgeons employ specialized imaging devices to capture this fluorescence, facilitating real-time visualization of parameters such as blood flow, tissue perfusion and lymphatic drainage [21]. The dynamic information garnered through ICG administration significantly augments intraoperative decision-making capabilities, enabling the meticulous assessment of vascular integrity, identification of viable tissues and optimization of procedural outcomes, particularly in flap reconstructions and microvascular or lymphatic surgeries [22]. The technique's non-invasive nature and swift clearance further bolster its safety profile and efficacy, underscoring its utility in guiding precise and sophisticated surgical interventions.

The aim of this article Is to contribute to the existing body of knowledge by providing a comprehensive review of the current literature while also introducing an innovative surgical approach for managing PNI. We hope that this article draws attention to the rather rare but also likely underdiagnosed condition of PNI [5], with special focus on the surgical treatment in cases of large PNI.

2. Methods

Ethics approval: The study was approved by Spital Thurgau HPC Research Committee. No additional approval of the Kanthonal Ethics Board (EKOS Ostschweiz) was sought for the following reasons: outcome analysis was performed retrospectively on anonymised patient data, no additional examination of patients was planned nor performed, no potential change of treatment was implied. The study was performed in accordance with the ethical standards laid down in the 1964 Declaration of Helsinki and its later amendments.

The literature review was performed by including all PubMed listed articles referring to the search term perineal nodular induration or cyclist's nodule published between 1990 and 2023. In particular, gender distribution and etiologic factors were reviewed, and the articles describing an operative procedure were analysed on surgical technique and outcome.

Presentation of our department's experience in the context of PNI: A 42-year-old, otherwise healthy, male presented to our department of plastic surgery upon referral from the department of urology with a 10-year history with a nodular perineal lesion. He reported a progression of the swelling over the years, with the development of a small, non-healing, secreting wound becoming prominent in the past few months. At the time of presentation at our department, he was road cycling between 10–15 h weekly on a semi-professional basis and felt increasingly impaired by the tissue proliferation. The patient denied any sensibility impairment, erectile dysfunction or dysuria. Physical examination revealed a 12 × 6 × 4.5 cm large, mobile, non-tender, partially fibrotic mound of perineal tissue. On the base of the tumor there was a 3 mm small, sharply demarcated, circular secreting ulceration (see Figure 1). Ultrasonography revealed a mass of hypoechoic tissue with singular hyperechoic lesions and sparse perfusion inferior to the raphe, with no testicular abnormalities. Native and contrast enhanced T2-weighted MRIs demonstrated a non-homogeneous soft tissue proliferation with unclear demarcation to the surroundings, which was classified as a diffuse, partially fibrotic tissue transformation (see Figure 2). The patient history and clinical findings pointed to the diagnosis of an extensive cyclist's nodule with fibrosis related disruption of lymphatic drainage. Considering the available literature and the size of the lesion, we recommended surgical excision with tissue doubling and optional lymph vessel obliteration assisted by intraoperative ICG-monitoring in inpatient setting.

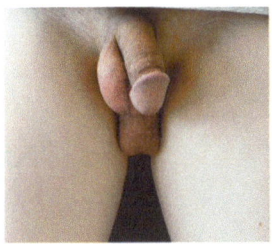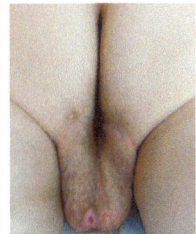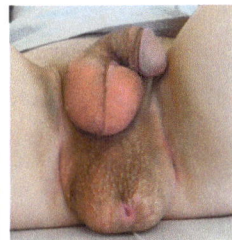

Figure 1. Clinical findings upon the first visit at our department of plastic surgery: The patient presented with a 12 × 6 × 4.5 cm large, mobile, non-tender, partially fibrotic mound of excess perineal tissue extending from the posterior base of the scrotum to the perianal area. On the base of the tumor, a small, circular, secreting ulceration could be seen that had only developed in the recent months.

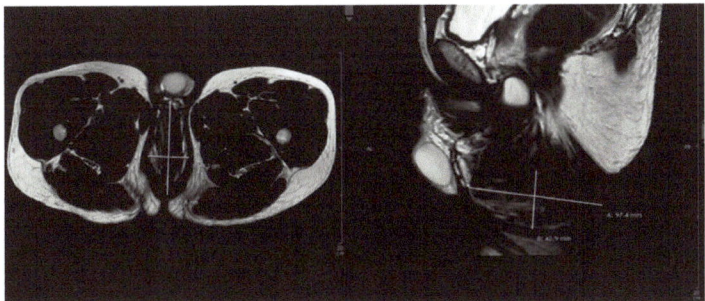

Figure 2. Diagnostic imaging: native and contrast enhanced T2-weighted MRI demonstrated a non-homogenous soft tissue proliferation with unclear demarcation to the surroundings, which was classified as a diffuse, partially fibrotic tissue transformation.

Surgical procedure: Surgery was performed under general anesthesia. The patient was placed in a lithotomy position. Perioperative antibiotic prophylaxis with amoxicillin/clavulanic acid was administered. The surgical procedure was performed under standard sterile conditions and surgical loupe magnification of ×2.5. The incision was marked, planning for a multiple W-plasty reaching from the apex, near the scrotum, down to 1 cm above the anus. Deepithelialization of a 3 cm wide dermal strip to the left of the planned incision was conducted before excision of the tumor. The tumor was dissected en bloc with overlying tissue under conservation of blood vessels, nerves and surrounding muscle (see Figure 3). The specimen was sent to the pathology department for histological examination. After this, 5 mL indocyanine green solution (VERDYE 5 mg/mL, Diagnostic Green GmbH, Germany) were subcutaneously injected bilateral into the proximal inner thigh for detection of lymphatic flow and possible leakages. With the help of the ICG handheld camera (IC-Flow™ Imaging System, Diagnostic Green GmbH, Germany), several small lymphatic vessels were identified and subsequently obliterated using bipolar cautery forceps (see Figure 4). Subtle thermic obliteration was performed for hemostasis before fitting a Redon drain (10 Charrière). The deepithelialized strip was placed underneath the opposing edge of the wound and fixed transcutaneously to provide a padding-effect by doubling the tissue. The overlying W-plasty was adapted and the skin closed via simple interrupted suture using Monocryl 4-0. Finally, a negative pressure wound therapy device was placed epicutaneously over the surgical wound, applying a continuous negative pressure of 125 mmHG.

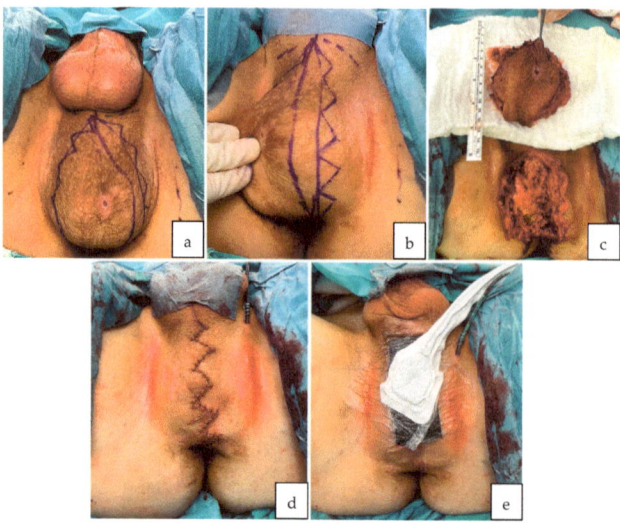

Figure 3. Step-by-step operative technique: (**a,b**) The patient was placed in a lithotomy position. The incision was marked, planning for a multiple W-plasty reaching from the apex, near the scrotum, down to 1 cm above the anus. (**c**) After deepithelialization of a 3 cm wide dermal strip to the left of the planned incision, the tumor was dissected en bloc with overlying tissue under conservation of blood vessels, nerves and surrounding muscle. (**d**) After hemostasis and obliteration of lymphatic leakages, a Redon drain (10 Charrière) was inserted before placing the deepithelialized strip underneath the opposing edge of the wound and fixing it transcutaneously to provide a padding-effect by doubling the tissue. The overlying W-plasty was adapted, and the skin was closed via simple interrupted suture. (**e**) A negative pressure wound therapy device was placed epicutaneously over the surgical wound, applying a continuous negative pressure of 125 mmHG.

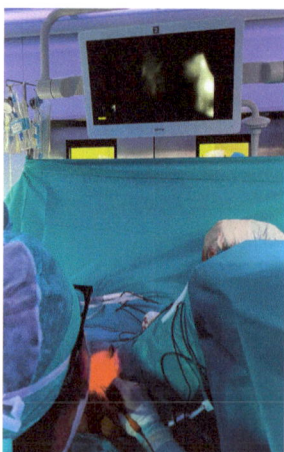

Figure 4. ICG imaging: 5 mL indocyanine green solution (VERDYE 5 mg/mL, Diagnostic Green GmbH, Germany) were injected subcutaneously bilaterally into the proximal inner thigh. An ICG handheld camera (IC-Flow™ Imaging System, Diagnostic Green GmbH, Germany) was used to detect lymphatic flow and possible leakages, which were subsequently obliterated using bipolar cautery forceps.

3. Results

The literature research yielded 16 PubMed articles encompassing 23 cases of perineal nodular induration (PNI) or cyclist's nodule. Of these, 9 cases involved females, and 14 involved males. Conservative treatment was documented in 7 cases (30%), while surgical approaches were reported in 16 cases (70%). Notably, a limited number of articles focused on histopathological or radiological characteristics, with a shortage of structured reviews on surgical treatment options. Only two articles provided detailed insights into surgical techniques.

Our patient's recovery after the procedure was prompt and without complications. He mobilized on the next day and reported no pain under standard analgesic therapy with NSAIDs and paracetamol. The drain and vacuum dressing were removed upon dismissal two days after the surgery. The perioperative antibiotic prophylaxis with amoxicillin/clavulanic acid was continued for a total of five days after surgery. Early postoperative recommendations consisted of sexual abstinence, no bathing, and daily dressing changes for two weeks.

Macroscopically the histopathological specimen consisted of skin and subcutaneous tissue, weighing 63 g. On the surface, there was a central, scarred ulcus measuring 1×1.2 cm. The cutting surface was inhomogeneous, white and soft with no clear demarcation of a focus border. Microscopically, the deeper tissues showed soft tissue collagen bundles mixed with fibroblasts, vessels and fat tissue. Focally, cystic degeneration was noted, but with no indication of a lymphocele or malignancy.

The patient was seen in our outpatient clinic electively one day after dismissal, and then two weeks, six weeks, six months and twelve months post-operatively. The wound healed uneventfully. At six weeks post-surgery, the patient reported reuptake of cycling without discomfort and still no issues with pain, sensibility impairment, erectile dysfunction or dysuria. Figure 5 shows the patient's perineum and scrotum at the two week, six week and six month follow-up with regular wound healing, minimal scar tissue formation (Vancouver scar scale 0) and no signs of a residual mass tissue. Ultrasound examination six months post-surgery showed neither fluid collection in the sense of oedema nor signs of recurrence (Figure 5).

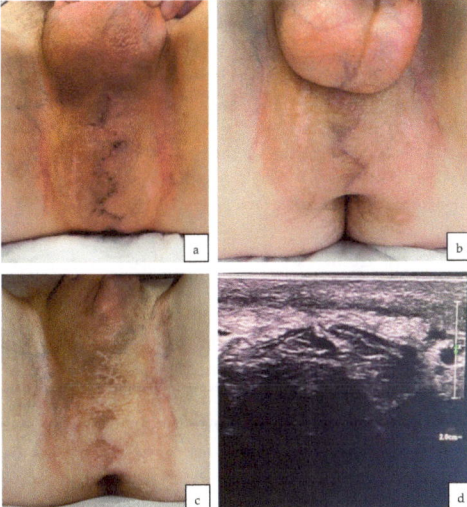

Figure 5. Clinical presentation of the surgical site at various follow-up visits: (**a**) Two weeks post-surgery showing regular wound healing, (**b**) six weeks post-surgery and (**c**) six months post-surgery showing minimal scar tissue formation (Vancouver scar scale) and no signs of a residual mass tissue. (**d**) The ultrasound at six months showed no sign of recurrence.

4. Discussion

Pathogenesis of PNI is attributed to the repetitive contact between the saddle and ischial tuberosities, and friction of the superficial perineal fascia against bony structures is thought to cause local injury, resulting in reparative proliferation of fibroblasts and myofibroblasts [3,4]. Chronic lymphedema resulting in the development of fibrous tissue has also been suggested as an etiological pathway of PNI [4]. Histopathological findings vary but tend to show necrosis of the superficial perineal fascia with myxoid degeneration of collagen fibers and fatty tissue, as well as occasional formation of a central pseudocyst [2–5,12,15]. In large PNIs, the skin condition with non-healing, exuding wounds often resembles other lymphatic problems, such as elephantiasis.

Clinical differential diagnoses vary in their likelihood depending on the patient's age and sex. Common causes of perineal nodular lesions include hydrocoeles, varicoceles [23], lymph nodes, herniae, aneurysms [6] and various neoplasms, such as angiomyofibroblastoma (AMF)-like tumors and aggressive angiomyofibroblastoma [13,24]. Histopathologically, the central pseudocyst may resemble ischemic fasciitis, as seen in elderly patients with bony protuberances [2]. Due to the low number of published cases of PNI (namely the 23 PubMed listed between 1990 and 2023), it can be assumed that PNI is a relatively rare disease; however, no statement can be made regarding the absolute prevalence. Furthermore, the low number of published cases is also the reason why no significant difference in the gender-specific prevalence should be made, even though more case reports on male patients than on female patients have been published.

In most cases, typical patient history, localization, and appearance during physical examination can diagnose PNI. Additionally, imaging modalities, such as ultrasound and magnetic resonance imaging, can be used as non-invasive techniques to secure a diagnosis [13]. An algorithm published by Norman et al. in a case report in 2020 may also help reach a diagnosis in unclear cases [5].

In our hands, the diagnosis of PNI was formed based on the patient's cycling history, clinical examination, as well as US and MRI imaging.

Conservative treatment options that have been discussed include a reduction in cycling activity [3,6] and saddle adjustments, ranging from substituting a dome-shaped saddle with a flatter one to a cutout or channel through the middle of the saddle [5]. In cases where bike and saddle fit have already been maximized, and where a reduction in activity is unrealistic (such as in professional cyclists), intralesional corticosteroid or hyaluronidase injections may provide relief [3,16,19,20]. However, steroid injections are solely recommended for small to medium sized lesions due to the risk of subcutaneous atrophy [3].

Recently published cases of the results of conservative treatment of similar lesions have reported that the lesions remained stable for a period of 5 months [6] and 1 year [13] after a reduction in cycling activity and readjusting saddle fitting conditions.

However, a "steady state" is not in the interest of most patients due to the size of the lesion and the significant impairment it causes.

Surgical excision has been suggested as the treatment of choice in cases refractory to conservative treatment [2,16,19].

Then again, other authors have advised against the surgical removal of these lesions due the risk of recurrence and the potentially irritating nature of the resulting scar tissue [3]. Additionally, the role of lymphatic drainage in PNI also remains controversial.

Based on our experience, we consider at least lymphatic impairment to be the main cause of the progression of a PNI. If, for example, a clinical picture of a PNI is compared with that of a penoscrotal lymphedema (PL), there is a striking similarity [24]. A recently published paper describes how, in advanced PL, surgical resection and penoscrotal reconstruction is the treatment of choice. In addition, Ehrl et al. suggest vascularized lymph node transfer (VLNT) to the groin or scrotum to be considered to improve the long-term surgical outcome in the sense of causal recurrence prophylaxis [25,26]. VLNT in general represents a surgical intervention for the management of lymphedeme. The procedure involves the extraction of healthy lymph nodes, typically sourced from the armpit or inguinal region, along with their associated vasculature. Employing precise microsurgical techniques, these nodes are intricately anastomosed to blood vessels at the targeted recipient site. Postoperatively, patients undergo a regimen of rehabilitation to optimize functional outcomes. Systematic follow-up assessments are imperative to evaluating the progression of the transplant's efficacy. This nuanced surgical approach endeavors to ameliorate lymphatic drainage, mitigating edema and enhancing the overall quality of life [27]. In our surgical therapeutic approach to late-stage PNI, VLNT has not yet been an adjuvant treatment option, but may be discussed in cases of recurrence despite a previous elaborate surgical approach.

The clinical picture of the pronounced PNI clearly implied a lymphatic drainage problem. We decided to address the lymphedema/leakage issue using ICG-assisted intraoperative lymph vessel obliteration in addition to tissue doubling and W-plasty-designed incisions to prevent tension, as well as epicutaneous negative wound dressing.

The application of ICG is clinically well-established in the evaluation of tissue perfusion within the context of free flaps [21]. Furthermore, the ICG camera is used as an adjunctive method for the visualization of lymphatic flow and, lately, for the detection of sentinel lymph nodes [28,29]. ICG diagnostic agents involve non-ionizing radiation, and side-effects are rarely seen. The ICG handheld camera can help to identify lymphatic vessels intraoperatively, and it also allows the surgeon to obliterate lymphatic leakage upon detection.

Due to the wound's localization in an area where bacterial contamination from the anogenital tract is likely [30], we decided to protect it by using an epicutaneous negative wound therapy device for the first two postoperative days. The device reduces tension in the suture area and can prevent surgical site infections [11]. This kind of wound dressing proved to be comfortable both for the surgeon and the patient.

Comparing our surgical approach with alternative methods described in the literature, particularly in the context of PNI, is challenging due to the scarcity of studies directly comparing outcomes. Two other studies shed light on different surgical techniques for PNI, allowing for a preliminary exploration of comparative considerations.

Awad et al. presented a surgical excision approach involving a spindle-shaped mass excision and wound closure by bilateral advancement flaps [2]. In contrast, Peters et al. described an incision at the lateral side of the perineum, resection of the mass and simple wound closure [16]. These approaches provide valuable insights into the diversity of surgical strategies employed in managing PNI.

This article highlights the relevance to the various disciplines involved in the diagnostics and treatment of PNI, and it is the first to describe the use of intraoperative ICG visualization and the application of an epicutaneous negative wound therapy device in this context. This novel therapeutic strategy proved successful with the patient's full return to health and no recurrence over the observation period of 12 months.

5. Conclusions

Surgical excision combined with W-shaped tissue doubling, lymph vessel obliteration assisted by intraoperative ICG visualization and postoperative epicutaneous negative wound dressing proved to be a successful treatment strategy for large PNI. The application of ICG and epicutaneous negative therapy has not been described in the context of PNI treatment so far. Based on the presumed context of lymphatic congestion in PNI, we believe that ICG visualization can result in minimizing the risk of developing a postoperative lymphocele and the overall risk of recurrence.

However, it is essential to clarify that the conclusions drawn are primarily descriptive in nature. The uniqueness of our innovative surgical technique is presented, aiming to contribute to the evolving landscape of PNI treatment options.

Due to the limited availability of studies directly comparing outcomes across various surgical procedures and postoperative regimens for PNI, our discussion leans towards providing a detailed account of our approach rather than offering definitive conclusions regarding its superiority over alternative methods.

Furthermore, we acknowledge the need for further research and comparative studies involving larger cohorts to comprehensively evaluate the efficacy and recurrence rates associated with different surgical interventions and postoperative care protocols.

Author Contributions: Conceptualization J.M.M., S.I.S. and T.H.; methodology J.M.M., S.I.S., C.K.M. and T.H.; formal analysis J.M.M., S.I.S., C.K.M., R.L., C.Z. and T.H.; investigation J.M.M. and T.H.; data curation J.M.M., S.I.S. and T.H.; writing—original draft preparation J.M.M., S.I.S., C.K.M. and T.H.; writing—review and editing J.M.M., S.I.S., C.K.M., C.Z. and T.H.; visualization J.M.M. and S.I.S. All authors have read and agreed to the published version of the manuscript.

Funding: This research received no external funding.

Institutional Review Board Statement: The study was conducted in accordance with the Declaration of Helsinki.

Informed Consent Statement: Written informed consent has been obtained from the patient to publish this paper.

Data Availability Statement: Supporting data are available from the authors upon request.

Conflicts of Interest: The authors declare no conflicts of interest.

References

1. Gonzalez-Perez, R.; Carneroa, L.; Arbide, N.; Soloeta, R. Perineal nodular induration in cyclists. *Actas Dermosifiliogr.* **2009**, *100*, 919–920. [CrossRef]
2. Awad, M.A.; Murphy, G.P.; Gaither, T.W.; Osterberg, E.C.; Sanford, T.A.; Horvai, A.E.; Breyer, B.N. Surgical excision of perineal nodular induration: A cyclist's third testicle. *Can. Urol. Assoc. J.* **2017**, *11*, E244–E247. [CrossRef] [PubMed]
3. Köhler, P.; Utermann, S.; Kahle, B.; Hartschuh, W. "Biker's nodule"– die perineale knotige Induration des Radsportlers. *Der Hautarzt* **2000**, *51*, 763–765. [CrossRef]
4. McCluggage, W.G.; Smith, J.H. Reactive fibroblastic and myofibroblastic proliferation of the vulva (Cyclist's Nodule): A hitherto poorly described vulval lesion occurring in cyclists. *Am. J. Surg. Pathol.* **2011**, *35*, 110–114. [CrossRef]
5. Norman, M.; Vitale, K. "Bumpy" ride for the female cyclist: A rare case of perineal nodular induration, the ischial hygroma. *Int. J. Surg. Case Rep.* **2020**, *73*, 277–280. [CrossRef]
6. Stoneham, A.; Thway, K.; Messiou, C.; Smith, M. Cyclist's nodule: No smooth ride. *BMJ Case Rep.* **2016**, *2016*, bcr2015213087. [CrossRef]
7. Creff, A.; Melki, F.; Ceccaldi, M.; Aubert, Y. L'hygroma ischiatique ou "troisième testicule du stayer". Réflexion à propos de l'étiopathogénie, du traitement et de la prévention. *Med. Sport.* **1985**, *59*, 296–300.
8. Leibovitch, I.; Mor, Y. The vicious cycling: Bicycling related urogenital disorders. *Eur. Urol.* **2005**, *47*, 277–286; discussion 286–287. [CrossRef]
9. Baeyens, L.; Vermeersch, E.; Bourgeois, P. Bicyclist's vulva: Observational study. *Bmj* **2002**, *325*, 138–139. [CrossRef]
10. Egli, H.; Totschnig, L.; Samartzis, N.; Kalaitzopoulos, D.R. Biker's nodule in women: A case report and review of the literature. *Case Rep. Womens Health* **2023**, *39*, e00539. [CrossRef]
11. Norman, G.; Goh, E.L.; Dumville, J.C.; Shi, C.; Liu, Z.; Chiverton, L.; Stankiewicz, M.; Reid, A. Negative pressure wound therapy for surgical wounds healing by primary closure. *Cochrane Database Syst. Rev.* **2020**, *6*, Cd009261.
12. Khedaoui, R.; Martin-Fragueiro, L.M.; Tardio, J.C. Perineal nodular induration ("Biker's nodule"): Report of two cases with fine-needle aspiration cytology and immunohistochemical study. *Int. J. Surg. Pathol.* **2014**, *22*, 71–75. [CrossRef]
13. De Cima, A.; Perez, N.; Ayala, G. MR imaging findings in perineal nodular induration ("cyclist s nodule"): A case report. *Radiol. Case Rep.* **2020**, *15*, 1091–1094. [CrossRef]
14. Makhanya, N.Z.; Velleman, M.; Suleman, F.E. A case of cyclist's nodule in a female patient. *S. Afr. J. Sports Med.* **2014**, *26*, 93–94. [CrossRef]
15. Van de Perre, S.; Vanhoenacker, F.M.; Vanstraelen, L.; Gaens, J.; Michiels, M. Perineal nodular swelling in a recreational cyclist: Diagnosis and discussion. *Skeletal Radiol.* **2009**, *38*, 919–920, 933–934. [CrossRef] [PubMed]
16. Peters, K.T.; Luyten, P.; Monstrey, S. Biker's Nodule: A Case Report and Review of the Literature. *Acta Chir. Belg.* **2014**, *114*, 414–416. [CrossRef]
17. Devers, K.G.; Heckman, S.R.; Muller, C.; Joste, N.E. Perineal Nodular Induration: A Trauma-induced Mass in a Female Equestrian. *Int. J. Gynecol. Pathol.* **2010**, *29*, 398–401. [CrossRef]
18. O'Donnell, T.F., Jr.; Allison, G.M.; Iafrati, M.D. A systematic review of guidelines for lymphedema and the need for contemporary intersocietal guidelines for the management of lymphedema. *J. Vasc. Surg. Venous Lymphat. Disord.* **2020**, *8*, 676–684. [CrossRef]

19. Amer, T.; Thayaparan, A.; Tasleem, A.; Aboumarzouk, O.; Bleehen, R.; Jenkins, B. An avid cyclist presenting with a 'third testicle'. *J. Clin. Urol.* **2015**, *8*, 429–431. [CrossRef]
20. Pharis, D.B.; Teller, C.; Wolf, J.E., Jr. Cutaneous manifestations of sports participation. *J. Am. Acad. Dermatol.* **1997**, *36*, 448–459. [CrossRef]
21. Ludolph, I.; Horch, R.E.; Arkudas, A.; Schmitz, M. Enhancing Safety in Reconstructive Microsurgery Using Intraoperative Indocyanine Green Angiography. *Front. Surg.* **2019**, *6*, 39. [CrossRef]
22. Chao, A.H.; Schulz, S.A.; Povoski, S.P. The application of indocyanine green (ICG) and near-infrared (NIR) fluorescence imaging for assessment of the lymphatic system in reconstructive lymphaticovenular anastomosis surgery. *Expert. Rev. Med. Devices* **2021**, *18*, 367–374. [CrossRef]
23. Frauscher, F.; Klauser, A.; Stenzl, A.; Helweg, G.; Amort, B.; zur Nedden, D. US findings in the scrotum of extreme mountain bikers. *Radiology* **2001**, *219*, 427–431. [CrossRef] [PubMed]
24. McCluggage, W.G.; Patterson, A.; Maxwell, P. Aggressive angiomyxoma of pelvic parts exhibits oestrogen and progesterone receptor positivity. *J. Clin. Pathol.* **2000**, *53*, 603–605. [CrossRef] [PubMed]
25. Ehrl, D.; Heidekrueger, P.I.; Giunta, R.E.; Wachtel, N. Giant Penoscrotal Lymphedema-What to Do? Presentation of a Curative Treatment Algorithm. *J. Clin. Med.* **2023**, *12*, 7586. [CrossRef] [PubMed]
26. Ehrl, D.; Tritschler, S.; Haas, E.M.; Alhadlg, A.; Giunta, R.E. Skrotales Lymphödem. *Handchir. Mikrochir. Plast. Chir.* **2018**, *50*, 299–302. [CrossRef]
27. Schaverien, M.V.; Badash, I.; Patel, K.M.; Selber, J.C.; Cheng, M.H. Vascularized Lymph Node Transfer for Lymphedema. *Semin. Plast. Surg.* **2018**, *32*, 28–35. [CrossRef] [PubMed]
28. Burnier, P.; Niddam, J.; Bosc, R.; Hersant, B.; Meningaud, J.P. Indocyanine green applications in plastic surgery: A review of the literature. *J. Plast. Reconstr. Aesthet. Surg.* **2017**, *70*, 814–827. [CrossRef] [PubMed]
29. Nishigori, N.; Koyama, F.; Nakagawa, T.; Nakamura, S.; Ueda, T.; Inoue, T.; Kawasaki, K.; Obara, S.; Nakamoto, T.; Fujii, H.; et al. Visualization of Lymph/Blood Flow in Laparoscopic Colorectal Cancer Surgery by ICG Fluorescence Imaging (Lap-IGFI). *Ann. Surg. Oncol.* **2016**, *23* (Suppl. 2), S266–S274. [CrossRef] [PubMed]
30. Sharma, R.K.; Parashar, A. The management of perineal wounds. *Indian. J. Plast. Surg.* **2012**, *45*, 352–363.

Disclaimer/Publisher's Note: The statements, opinions and data contained in all publications are solely those of the individual author(s) and contributor(s) and not of MDPI and/or the editor(s). MDPI and/or the editor(s) disclaim responsibility for any injury to people or property resulting from any ideas, methods, instructions or products referred to in the content.

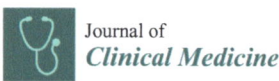 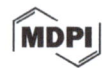

Article

PlasmaBlade versus Electrocautery for Deep Inferior Epigastric Perforator Flap Harvesting in Autologous Breast Reconstruction: A Comparative Clinical Outcome Study

Angela Augustin, Ines Schoberleitner, Sophie-Marie Unterhumer, Johanna Krapf, Thomas Bauer and Dolores Wolfram *

Department of Plastic, Reconstructive and Aesthetic Surgery, Medical University of Innsbruck, 6020 Innsbruck, Austria
* Correspondence: dolores.wolfram@i-med.ac.at; Tel.: +43-(0)-512-504-22731

Abstract: (1) **Background**: DIEP-based breast reconstruction necessitates wide undermining at the abdominal donor site, creating large wound areas. Flap harvesting is usually conducted using electrosurgical dissection devices. This study sought to compare the clinical outcomes in patients after using the PEAK PlasmaBlade (PPB) versus monopolar electrocautery (MPE). (2) **Methods**: This retrospective cohort study included 128 patients with DIEP-based breast reconstruction. Patient characteristics and information on the postoperative course were collected and a comparative evaluation was conducted. (3) **Results**: The MPE group exhibited significantly ($p^* = 0.0324$) higher abdominal drainage volume (351.11 ± 185.96 mL) compared to the PPB group (279.38 ± 183.38 mL). A subgroup analysis demonstrated that PPB significantly reduced postoperative wound fluid in patients with BMI > 30 kg/m^2 ($p^* = 0.0284$), without prior neoadjuvant chemotherapy ($p^{**} = 0.0041$), and among non-smokers ($p = 0.0046$). Furthermore, postoperative pain was significantly ($p^{****} < 0.0001$) lower in the PPB cohort. (4) **Conclusions**: This study confirms the non-inferiority of the PEAK PlasmaBlade to conventional electrocautery for abdominal flap harvesting. The PPB demonstrated advantages, notably reduced drainage volume and lower postoperative pain levels. Recognizing patient subsets that benefit more from the PPB highlights the importance of personalized device selection based on patient characteristics.

Keywords: autologous breast reconstruction; clinical outcome; electrosurgery; flap harvesting; PEAK PlasmaBlade

1. Introduction

Abdominal-based flaps, particularly the deep inferior epigastric perforator (DIEP) flap, have become the standard approach for autologous breast reconstruction following nipple-sparing mastectomy (NSME) or skin-sparing mastectomy (SSME) procedures [1–3]. This technique offers several notable advantages, including an enhanced quality of life and greater patient satisfaction when compared to implant-based approaches [4–6]. However, the trade-offs are longer surgical duration, extended hospital stay and the necessity to sacrifice an additional donor site. Considering this additional effort, our objective should be to minimize the risks associated with the additional surgery for the patients and continuously strive to enhance the surgical outcome.

Abdominal flap harvesting is performed with electrosurgical devices, using high-frequency electrical current for tissue dissection and simultaneous hemostasis [7]. Different modalities are available, the conventional monopolar electrocautery (MPE) uses a continuous waveform of radiofrequency energy via an uninsulated metal electrode for tissue cutting through thermal ablation, operating at temperatures between 180 and 240 °C [8]. In contrast, the PEAK PlasmaBlade (PPB) employs short (40 µs) high-frequency pulses of radiofrequency energy to generate electrical plasma along an insulated electrode's edge and it maintains a lower operating temperature around 45 °C [8,9]. Previous investigations suggest that the PlasmaBlade may offer advantages over electrocautery, demonstrating reduced thermal injury depth and inflammatory responses [8,10,11]. Inflammatory processes and trauma to the lymphatic network during surgical dissection are known factors contributing to postoperative seroma formation, a common complication after DIEP flap harvesting, with reported incidences ranging from 1.4% to 16.2% [12–16]. Prolonged drainage duration to prevent seroma formation poses disadvantages such as extended hospitalization and the risk of ascending infections through the drain tube. Previous research has generated conflicting and inconclusive findings regarding whether the choice of the surgical dissection device significantly impacts clinical outcomes. While some studies suggest benefits associated with using the PPB, such as reduced seroma rates and shorter drain dwelling times, these studies have limitations, notably small sample sizes and none have evaluated patient-specific risk factors in this context [11,17–22].

Our study seeks to evaluate the influence of the dissection device utilized during abdominal flap harvesting on clinical outcomes, while considering risk factors, such as body mass index (BMI), smoking status and previous chemotherapy.

2. Materials and Methods

This retrospective, single-center cohort study was approved by the Institutional Ethics Committee of Medical University Innsbruck (protocol code 1082/2021).

2.1. Patients

We included a total of 128 patients who underwent autologous DIEP flap breast reconstruction at our department between 2013 and 2020. Among these, 56 patients underwent abdominal flap harvesting using the PEAK PlasmaBlade (Medtronic, Dublin, Ireland) (PPB), while 72 patients underwent the procedure using monopolar electrocautery (MPE). Assignment to the surgical device was carried out chronologically. Initially, flap dissection with monopolar electrocautery was the standard procedure until the PEAK PlasmaBlade became consistently available at our department. Subsequently, the PPB replaced monopolar electrocautery as the standard dissection device. Inclusion criteria were defined as age over 18 years, uni- or bilateral NSME or SSME, and immediate or staged DIEP-based autologous breast reconstruction by or under the supervision of one single surgeon, who has been a senior member and specialized microsurgeon for over 10 years by the time of the first included patient in this study. To prevent bias, one patient was excluded due to the development of extreme seroma formation (1730 mL). In the case of the excluded patient, flap dissection was performed using monopolar electrocautery. This patient was a 73-year-old undergoing unilateral primary breast reconstruction with a BMI of 30.3 kg/m^2, non-smoker and without prior chemotherapy. Serous-sanguineous abdominal drainage fluid was highly elevated during the first 48 postoperative hours leading to revision under general anesthesia due to postoperative bleeding and a hematoma on the second postoperative day.

We conducted a retrospective chart analysis to assess patient demographics, complications and clinical outcomes. All patients included in this study underwent abdominal flap harvesting and received postoperative care following our institutional protocol. We made skin incisions using a steel scalpel and proceeded with subcutaneous tissue preparation using the electrosurgical device. Blood vessels were coagulated using isolated forceps and cautery. To ensure safe perforator identification and dissection, we did not leave fatty tissue on the central aspects of the fascia abdominalis within the flap harvesting area. Perforator vessels were dissected using scissors and bipolar cauterization or surgical clips for hemostasis. Following flap harvest, we mobilized the tissue above the umbilicus in the central area using the electrosurgical device until closure with mild to moderate tension was feasible, if necessary, extending the mobilization to the sub-xiphoid area. During this final step, a fatty layer was left over the fascia to prevent seroma formation. However, we did not mobilize the lateral abdomen to optimize perfusion of the remaining abdominal cutaneous and subcutaneous tissue. Redon drains were placed at the end of surgery, just before wound closure, and were placed under suction (Figure 1). Drain removal was undertaken when the output was less than 30 mL per 24 h. The volume of drainage fluid was recorded at 24 h intervals. All patients were required to wear an abdominal binder for a duration of six weeks following surgery.

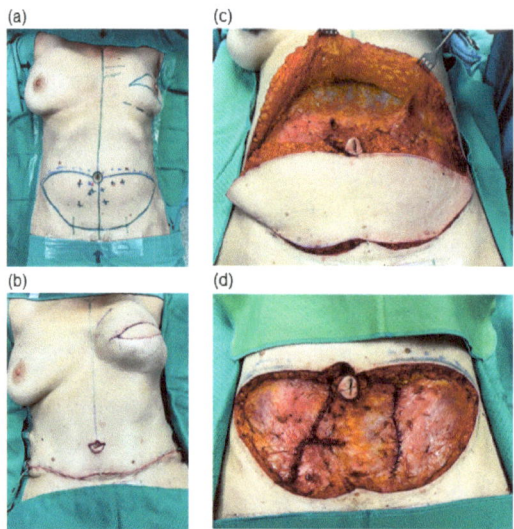

Figure 1. Intraoperative photo documentation of abdominal DIEP flap harvesting. (**a**) Preoperative markings of planned incisions. (**b**) Reconstructive result after skin-sparing mastectomy (resection weight: 650 g) on the left patient side and primary reconstruction (flap weight: 720 g). (**c**) Wound bed after mobilization, with the DIEP flap still in situ. (**d**) Defect after completion of DIEP flap harvesting (resection weight: 750 g).

For the PEAK PlasmaBlade, surgeries were conducted using standardized technical settings, with both the "cut" and "coagulate" functions set to intensity "6". These settings remained consistent across all patients, without individual adjustments. In the monopolar electrocautery group preferred settings were typically "cut" 40 W and "coagulation" 40 W. However, minor variations cannot be excluded due to incomplete documentation.

Postoperative pain levels were assessed at various time intervals within a 24 h period using the Numerical Analog Scale, which utilizes a scale ranging from 0 (indicating the absence of pain) to 10 (representing the most severe imaginable pain). If multiple values were recorded per day, the maximum daily score was included in the study.

2.2. Statistical Analysis

Statistical analysis was performed using Prism Software 10 for macOS (GraphPad Software, Boston, MA, USA) and Google Sheets (Google LLC, Mountain View, CA, USA; https://www.google.com/sheets/about/, accessed on 30 October 2023). To assess significant differences between the two groups, we employed the independent sample Student's *t*-test for continuous data. For categorical data, Fisher's exact and Chi-Square tests were utilized to determine statistical significance. A two-way analysis of variance (ANOVA) test was conducted to assess interactions between the types of surgical devices used (PPB versus MPE) and their individual effects on postoperative pain. Statistical significance of simple linear regression has been determined by comparison of slopes and intercepts with a confidence interval of 95%. A *p*-value of <0.05 was considered significant. The significance threshold was set at $p < 0.05$. The level for statistical significance was set at $p^{ns} \geq 0.05$, $p^* < 0.05$, $p^{**} < 0.02$, $p^{***} < 0.001$ and $p^{****} < 0.0001$ for all statistical tests.

3. Results

All 128 patients included in the study were categorized into two distinct cohorts based on the method employed for abdominal flap preparation: either utilizing the PEAK PlasmaBlade (PPB; $n = 56$) or the monopolar electrocautery (MPE; $n = 72$). An analysis of patient characteristics revealed no statistically significant distinctions between the two cohorts in terms of age, BMI, smoking status, neoadjuvant oncologic therapy, diabetes mellitus and the indication for mastectomy (Table 1).

Table 1. Patient characteristics.

	PPB	MPE	
n	56	72	
	Mean (±std)	Mean (±std)	p-Value
Age	49.68 (±10.50)	48.67 (±9.56)	0.5733
BMI	25.37 (±3.85)	25.33 (±4.01)	0.9612
Flap volume (mL)	617.16 (±283.66)	608.27 (±322.90)	0.8572
	n (%)	n%	p-value
Female	56 (100)	72 (100)	>0.999
Indication			
Carcinoma	53 (94.64)	71 (98.61)	0.2005
Prophylactic	3 (5.36)	1 (1.39)	
Breast reconstruction			
Unilateral	34 (60.7)	55 (76.4)	0.0560
Bilateral	22 (39.3)	17 (23.6)	
Nicotine			
Yes	6 (10.71)	12 (16.67)	0.3366
No	50 (89.29)	60 (83.33)	
Diabetes			
Yes	1 (1.79)	0 (0.00)	0.3918
No	55 (98.21)	72 (100.00)	
Neoadjuvant chemotherapy			
Yes	21 (37.50)	24 (33.33)	0.6243
No	35 (62.50)	48 (66.67)	
BMI			0.9692
BMI < 25 kg/m^2	32 (57.14)	40 (55.55)	
BMI 25–30 kg/m^2	15 (26.79)	21 (29.17)	
BMI > 30 kg/m^2	9 (16.07)	11 (15.28)	

Assessment of clinical outcomes through a comparative analysis between the two patient cohorts regarding the overall abdominal wound fluid production revealed a significantly ($p^* = 0.0324$) higher quantity within the monopolar electrocautery (MPE) group (351.11 ± 185.96 mL) in contrast to the PEAK PlasmaBlade (PPB) group (279.38 ± 183.38 mL) (Table 2 and Figure 2). An analysis of hospitalization duration (10.86 ± 2.29 days vs. 11.13 ± 3.00 days, $p^{ns} = 0.5828$) and drain dwell time (5.63 ± 1.54 days vs. 5.53 vs. 1.73 days, $p^{ns} = 0.6133$) demonstrated no significant discrepancies between the two patient cohorts.

Table 2. Clinical outcome.

	PPB	MPE	
Outcome	Mean (±std)	Mean (±std)	p-Value
Number of suction drainages	2.00 (±0.00)	1.99 (±0.12)	0.3799
Duration of draining (days)	6.18 (±1.69)	6.29 (±1.72)	0.7128
Hospitalization (days)	10.86 (±2.29)	11.13 (±3.00)	0.5828
Total wound fluid quantity (mL)	279.38 (±183.38)	351.11 (±185.96)	0.0324 *

Table 2. Cont.

Outcome	PPB Mean (±std)	MPE Mean (±std)	p-Value
Seroma (mL) and risk factors			
Non-Smoker	267.10 (±164.21)	367.92 (±195.73)	0.0046 **
Smoker	381.67 (±313.52)	267.08 (±107.84)	0.2612
Adjuvant Chemotherapy	325.00 (±215.56)	326.04 (±209.19)	0.9870
No Chemotherapy	252.00 (±161.23)	363.65 (±176.29)	0.0041 **
BMI < 25 kg/m^2	256.41 (±186.32)	315.25 (±175.01)	0.1727
BMI 25–30 kg/m^2	303.33 (±206.08)	335.95 (±168.64)	0.6053
BMI > 30 kg/m^2	321.11 (±146.33)	510.45 (±197.74)	0.0284 *

The level for statistical significance was set at * $p < 0.05$, ** $p < 0.02$.

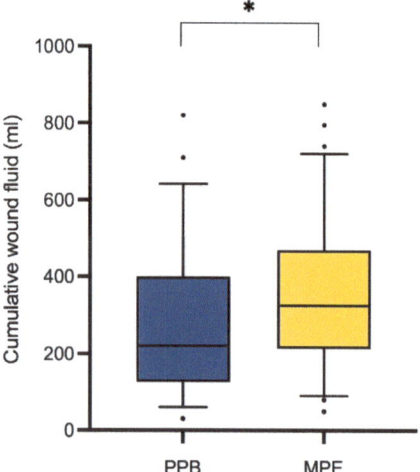

Figure 2. Cumulative postoperative wound fluid quantity (mL). Comparative analysis through Student's *t*-test indicates a significant increase ($p^* = 0.0324$) in the MPE cohort ($n = 72$) compared to the PPB cohort ($n = 56$).

3.1. Risk Factors

To evaluate the potential impact of various risk factors, patients were subdivided into specific groups based on their individual characteristics, followed by a comparison. Notably, a significant reduction in postoperative abdominal wound fluid production after surgery with the PPB was observed for non-smokers ($p^{**} = 0.0046$), those without prior neoadjuvant chemotherapy ($p^{**} = 0.0041$) and those with a BMI exceeding 30 kg/m^2 ($p^* = 0.0284$) (Table 2 and Figure 3).

To assess the relationship between BMI and wound fluid production, simple linear regression analysis was conducted (Figure 4). In the MPE cohort, a significant association emerged between higher BMI and increased postoperative wound fluid production ($p^{**} = 0.0058$). However, such a correlation was not observed within the PPB cohort ($p^{ns} = 0.2895$).

Within all subgroups that exhibited favorable outcomes associated with the use of PEAK PlasmaBlade (PPB) in the context of the volume of postoperative drainage fluid, an examination of both drain dwell time and the duration of hospitalization was performed. Consistent with the observed reduction in wound fluid volume, a tendency towards decreased drain dwell time and shortened hospital stays was observed, although these trends did not achieve statistical significance (Table 3).

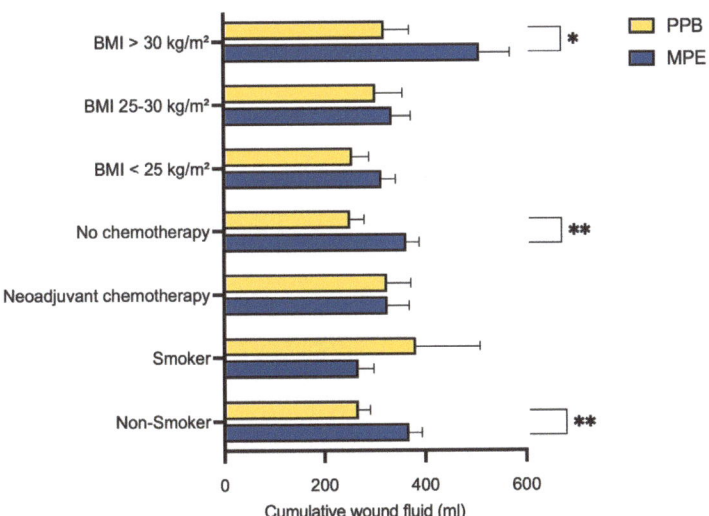

Figure 3. Evaluation of cumulative wound fluid quantity and risk factors. Mean and SEM of postoperative drainage volume (mL) are shown for both cohorts. Statistical significance was determined by Student's t-test, revealing a significant reduction in postoperative wound fluid production after surgery with the PPB for those with a BMI exceeding 30 kg/m^2 ($p^* = 0.0284$), those without prior neoadjuvant chemotherapy ($p^{**} = 0.0041$) and for non-smokers ($p^{**} = 0.0046$). The level for statistical significance was set at * $p < 0.05$, ** $p < 0.02$.

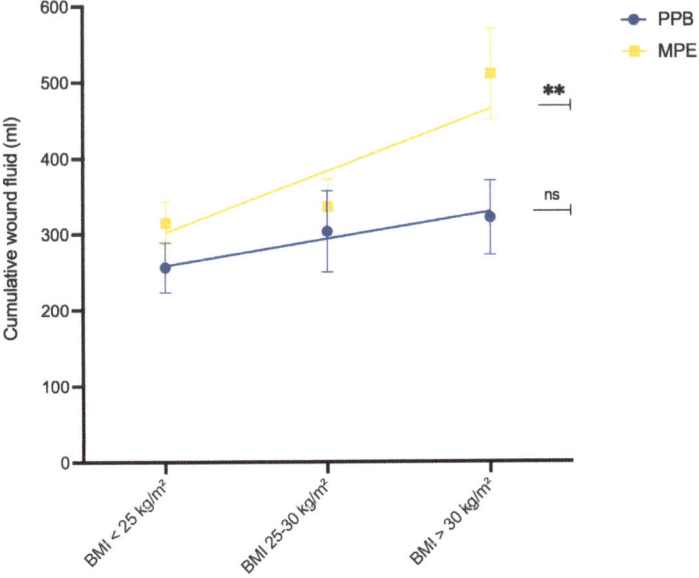

Figure 4. Relationship between BMI and wound fluid quantity (mL). In both groups, we compared the correlation of cumulative wound fluid quantity (mL) and BMI class by simple linear regression analysis. The analysis revealed a significant correlation between higher BMI class and increased postoperative wound fluid production in the MPE cohort. Slope significantly non-zero [PPB]: $F(1.54) = 1.144$, $p^{ns} = 0.2895$, $y = 35.19x + 223.4$; [MPE]: $F(1.70) = 8.104$, $p^{**} = 0.0058$, $y = 81.06x + 221.6$. The level for statistical significance was set at $^{ns} p \geq 0.05$, ** $p < 0.02$.

Table 3. Evaluation of drain dwell time and hospitalization within subgroups.

	PPB	MPE	
Drain Dwelling Time (d)	Mean (±std)	Mean (±std)	p-Value
Non-Smoker	6.10 (±1.50)	6.35 (±1.71)	0.4210
No chemotherapy	6.09 (±1.50)	6.35 (±1.62)	0.4440
BMI > 30 kg/m²	6.67 (±1.87)	7.55 (±1.75)	0.2933
Hospitalization (d)			
Non-Smoker	10.86 (±2.35)	11.00 (±2.26)	0.7513
No chemotherapy	10.94 (±2.71)	11.02 (±3.22)	0.9077
BMI > 30 kg/m²	11.44 (±4.03)	11.73 (±1.19)	0.8267

In the cohort of patients undergoing unilateral reconstruction, a noteworthy decrease in postoperative drainage fluid is observed in the PEAK PlasmaBlade group compared to monopolar electrocautery (p^{**} = 0.0077). Conversely, there is no statistically significant disparity between the two devices in bilateral reconstruction cases (p^{ns} = 0.9404). Additionally, when comparing unilateral and bilateral reconstructions irrespective of the surgical device, there is no noticeable difference in postoperative wound fluid quantity (p^{ns} = 0.7118) (Table 4).

Table 4. Evaluation of cumulative abdominal wound fluid quantity (mL) in uni- and bilateral breast reconstruction.

	PPB	MPE	
	Mean (±std)	Mean (±std)	p-Value
Unilateral	248.53 (±177.81)	357.09 (±184.89)	0.0077 **
Bilateral	327.05 (±189.92)	331.76 (±199.31)	0.9404
	Unilateral reconstruction	Bilateral reconstruction	
	mean (±std)	mean (±std)	p-value
All patients (n = 128)	315.62 (±188.80)	329.10 (±191.48)	0.7118

The level for statistical significance was set at ** p < 0.02.

3.2. Postoperative Complications and Pain

An analysis of postoperative complications did not yield any statistically significant distinctions between the two patient cohorts, both in terms of overall complications (p^{ns} = 0.2758) and in the specific assessment of bleeding or hematoma (p^{ns} = 0.7128) (Table 5). All postoperative complications, as per the Clavien–Dindo [23] classification, are outlined in Table 5.

Postoperative pain assessment was conducted using a Numerical Analog Scale, graded on a scale ranging from 0 (indicating no pain) to 10 (reflecting the most severe imaginable pain). As outlined in Table 6 and Figure 5, a comparative investigation between the two patient cohorts unveiled a statistically significant decrease in postoperative pain within the PPB group (p^{****} < 0.0001).

As depicted in Figure 5, postoperative pain rates decreased within both studied cohorts throughout the 10-day postoperative period. We compared postoperative pain levels on day 1 versus day 10 for both patient cohorts using a Student's t-test. This analysis revealed a significant decrease in pain levels in the PPB cohort (p^{**} = 0.0067), indicating a notable reduction in pain over time. However, in the MPE cohort, while there was a decrease in postoperative pain levels between day 1 and day 10, the t-test did not show significance (p^{ns} = 0.4071).

Table 5. Postoperative complications.

	PPB	MPE	
	n (%)	*n*%	*p*-Value
Complications	13 (23.21)	23 (31.94)	0.2758
Bleeding/Hematoma	4 (7.14)	4 (5.56)	0.7128
Clavien–Dindo			
1	5 (8.93)	10 (13.89)	
Bleeding/Hematoma	2 (3.57)	1 (1.39)	
Wound healing complications	3 (5.36)	7 (9.72)	
Seroma	0 (0.00)	2 (2.78)	
2	0 (0.00)	0 (0.00)	
3a	0 (0.00)	2 (2.78)	
Wound healing complications	0 (0.00)	2 (2.78)	
3b	8 (14.29)	11 (15.28)	
Bleeding/Hematoma	2 (3.57)	3 (4.17)	
Wound healing complications	6 (10.71)	8 (11.11)	

Table 6. Postoperative pain, Numerical Analog Scale (NAS) (0–10).

	PPB	MPE	
	Mean (±std)	Mean (±std)	*p*-Value
Day 1	2.36 (±1.52)	2.00 (±1.81)	0.4994
Day 2	2.23 (±1.47)	3.09 (±1.73)	0.0080 **
Day 3	2.08 (±1.62)	2.67 (±1.71)	0.0683
Day 4	1.71 (±1.18)	2.27 (±1.70)	0.0512
Day 5	1.73 (±1.59)	1.65 (±1.50)	0.7855
Day 6	1.29 (±1.12)	1.82 (±1.87)	0.0729
Day 7	0.88 (±0.93)	1.55 (±1.52)	0.0065 **
Day 8	1.27 (±1.35)	1.49 (±1.66)	0.4455
Day 9	1.07 (±1.18)	1.89 (±1.78)	0.0153 **
Day 10	1.23 (±1.34)	1.61 (±1.48)	0.2928

The level for statistical significance was set at ** $p < 0.02$.

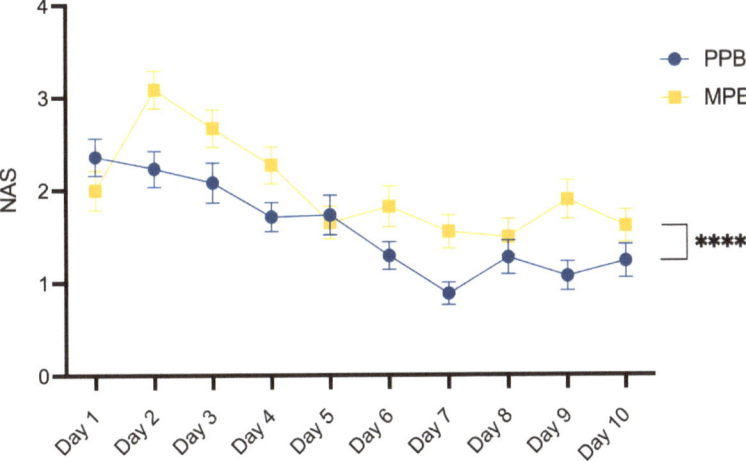

Figure 5. Comparative evaluation of postoperative pain. Mean and SEM for Numeric Analog Scale (NAS) assessment over a 10-day postoperative period. Statistical significance was determined by 2-way ANOVA: $p^{****} < 0.0001$, demonstrating a notable reduction in postoperative pain within the PEAK PlasmaBlade (PPB) group.

4. Discussion

Autologous DIEP-based breast reconstruction involves extensive undermining at the abdominal donor site, resulting in sizable wound areas. Typically, flap dissection is undertaken with electrosurgical devices to allow simultaneous hemostasis and efficient operating times [24]. We evaluated two specific dissection devices—the standard monopolar electrocautery and the newer PEAK PlasmaBlade—in the context of abdominal flap harvesting, aiming to discern their impacts on clinical outcomes.

Previous research has yielded conflicting and inconclusive results regarding whether the selection of the dissection device can genuinely lead to better clinical outcomes.

Studies assessing outcomes in extensive wound areas, like those involved in autologous breast reconstruction using the abdominal donor site, have often been limited by small sample sizes [11,17–22,25,26]. While more extensive investigations have been undertaken in distinct surgical contexts, such as tonsillectomy [27–29] and surgical implant replacement [30], these findings may not be directly applicable to the specific circumstances of autologous breast reconstruction.

Our retrospective analysis sought to broaden the scope of this research by including a total of 128 patients in our study. Of these patients, 72 underwent abdominal flap preparation using conventional electrocautery, while 56 patients underwent the procedure with the PEAK PlasmaBlade. A comparison of these two patient cohorts revealed no statistically significant differences in age, body mass index, smoking status, history of neoadjuvant oncologic therapy, diabetes status and the primary indication for mastectomy. This comparability ensures the reliability and robustness of our observed outcomes.

Our analysis yielded the significant ($p^* = 0.0324$) finding of a higher cumulative wound fluid quantity in the monopolar electrocautery group (351.11 ± 185.96 mL) compared to the PEAK PlasmaBlade group (279.38 ± 183.38 mL). While previous research on this topic has provided inconclusive data, some studies support our finding by reporting lower total drain output following the use of the PEAK PlasmaBlade [11,17–20,22], whereas other authors found no difference between the two dissection devices [21,25,26]. It is worth noting that, to the best of our knowledge, no prior study has reported an increase in seroma rates after utilizing the PEAK PlasmaBlade. It has previously been suggested that the reduced working temperature of the PEAK PlasmaBlade leads to lower tissue damage [8,10], which contributes to reduced seroma formation. One study in gender-affirming mastectomy patients has investigated histologic samples, showing a 22% reduction in thermal injury depth with the PlasmaBlade compared to conventional monopolar cautery [18].

Similarly, the existing literature on the evaluation of hospitalization and drain dwell time yields inconsistent results. While Schlosshauer, Dogan and Sowa reported positive outcomes in the PlasmaBlade cohorts [11,17,19,20], other studies did not identify variations in terms of hospitalization and drain dwell time [21,25,26]. Our data did not reveal a difference between both devices for these aspects. There is no previous work indicating inferiority of the PlasmaBlade in this regard.

We intentionally selected abdominal-based autologous breast reconstruction as our research focus. This patient group not only represents a highly standardized approach to large-scale wound preparation but also encompasses a spectrum of patient-specific risk factors, including those related to oncologic treatments, which are pertinent to our analysis. Extensive cohort studies conducted so far have failed to establish a definitive link between neoadjuvant chemotherapy and the occurrence of surgical complications during breast reconstruction [31–35]. Nevertheless, we were determined to assess the role of dissection instruments in relation to neoadjuvant chemotherapy and other risk factors and its impact on surgical outcomes. We identified chemotherapy, smoking status and BMI as the primary risk factors of interest in our patient cohorts, with prevalences high enough to enable statistical analysis.

In our multivariate data analysis, we identified a substantial reduction in postoperative abdominal wound fluid production in the PEAK PlasmaBlade cohort compared to the electrocautery cohort across three specific subgroups. These groups comprised individuals without prior neoadjuvant chemotherapy (p^{**} = 0.0041), non-smokers (p^{**} = 0.0046) and those with a BMI exceeding 30 kg/m^2 (p^* = 0.0284).

It is noteworthy that these groups typically do not share the same risk profile. In standard practice, non-smokers and patients without previous neoadjuvant chemotherapy are typically regarded as low-risk individuals for surgical complications. Conversely, patients with a BMI exceeding 30 kg/m^2 are commonly perceived as a high-risk population for adverse events in the surgical context [36]. Mani et al. previously investigated the association between BMI and the occurrence of donor-site seroma following the harvesting of DIEP flaps. Their findings revealed that obese patients (BMI > 30 kg/m^2) had the highest incidence of postoperative seroma formation, reaching a rate of 16% [16]. Our results revealed a significant association between higher BMI and increased postoperative wound fluid production (p^{**} = 0.0058) within the MPE cohort (Figure 4). In contrast, no such correlation was evident within the PPB cohort (p^{ns} = 0.2895), suggesting that the utilization of PPB might mitigate the risks associated with higher BMI.

Although not statistically significant, all subgroups that displayed positive outcomes with the use of the PEAK PlasmaBlade regarding postoperative drainage volume also demonstrated a trend toward reduced drain dwell time and shorter hospital stays.

The assessment of hospitalization duration may be subject to some inaccuracies, as our department typically retains patients in the hospital until histopathological results become accessible, and the removal of the monitoring skin island is performed. Nevertheless, it is noteworthy that a tendency towards reduced drainage catheter dwell time in the PPB group may potentially be linked to our observed outcomes of a significant decrease in postoperative pain levels around day 7 and day 9 in the PPB group, attributable to the earlier removal of drainage devices.

Our data reveal a significant decrease in postoperative pain within the PEAK PlasmaBlade cohort. To our knowledge, only Friebel et al. have previously compared postoperative pain levels between both dissection devices, reporting an increase in the PPB cohort [21]. This was attributed to the potential impact of tighter abdominal closure due to lower flap weights in this group. In our patient cohorts, both flap volume (p = 0.8572) and the distribution of unilateral versus bilateral reconstruction (p = 0.0560) within the two patient groups were comparable, as an analysis of our patient characteristics (Table 1) showed. We consider this as a strength of our study since it allows the assumption that postoperative pain levels are not biased by these characteristics. There have been studies examining postoperative pain following surgical skin incisions made with electrocautery versus steel scalpel, which reported reduced pain levels and a decreased use of analgesics in the electrocautery group [37,38]. Chrysos explains this by highlighting that the vaporization of cells resulting from the application of pure sinusoidal current leads to immediate tissue and nerve necrosis without significantly affecting nearby structures [38]. The varying degrees of nerve damage between electrocautery and the PEAK PlasmaBlade may also contribute to our significant finding of reduced postoperative pain in the PPB group, but such evaluations should be a focus of future studies.

Our study demonstrates also several limitations. Due to retrospective data analysis, we cannot offer detailed information concerning the adjustments of the used monopolar electrocautery. But we tried to overcome this lack of information by only including patients that were operated under the lead of one single surgeon, so it may be assumed that the same preferred settings were used. Furthermore, this study benefits from the extensive experience of this single surgeon, contributing to the reliability of the findings and minimizing the risk of performance bias. Moreover, the similarity in patient demographic characteristics across both cohorts indicates a low risk of selection bias, despite the study's retrospective nature.

5. Conclusions

In conclusion, our findings align with previous research, indicating that the PEAK PlasmaBlade is not inferior to conventional electrocautery. Furthermore, patients may experience advantages such as reduced drainage volume and lower postoperative pain levels following wound preparation with the PlasmaBlade. Notably, our analysis identified patient subgroups that could derive even greater benefits from the use of this device. In these specific patient groups, utilizing the PEAK PlasmaBlade could result in better clinical outcomes. Therefore, the choice to use this device may be based on the potential benefits for patients, rather than solely on the surgeon's subjective preferences.

Author Contributions: Conceptualization, D.W. and T.B.; methodology, T.B.; software, A.A. and I.S.; validation, A.A., J.K., I.S. and S.-M.U.; formal analysis, A.A.; investigation, T.B.; data curation, J.K. and S.-M.U.; writing—original draft preparation, A.A.; writing—review and editing, I.S. and D.W.; visualization, A.A.; supervision, D.W.; project administration, D.W., I.S. and T.B. All authors have read and agreed to the published version of the manuscript.

Funding: This research received no external funding.

Institutional Review Board Statement: The study was conducted in accordance with the Declaration of Helsinki, and approved by the Institutional Ethics Committee of MEDICAL UNIVERSITY INNSBRUCK (protocol code 1082/2021, 23 June 2021).

Informed Consent Statement: Written informed consent has been obtained from the patient to publish this paper.

Data Availability Statement: The data presented in this study are available on request from the corresponding author.

Acknowledgments: Stephan Sigl is acknowledged for providing clinical guidance and administrative support. The authors thank Karin Langert, Angelika Feichter and Theresa Zagrajsek for photo documentation of our patients.

Conflicts of Interest: The authors declare no conflicts of interest.

References

1. Allen, R.J.; Treece, P. Deep Inferior Epigastric Perforator Flap for Breast Reconstruction. *Ann. Plast. Surg.* **1994**, *32*, 32–38. [CrossRef] [PubMed]
2. Healy, C.; Allen, R.J. The Evolution of Perforator Flap Breast Reconstruction: Twenty Years after the First DIEP Flap. *J. Reconstr. Microsurg.* **2014**, *30*, 121–126. [CrossRef] [PubMed]
3. Granzow, J.W.; Levine, J.L.; Chiu, E.S.; Allen, R.J. Breast Reconstruction with the Deep Inferior Epigastric Perforator Flap: History and an Update on Current Technique. *J. Plast. Reconstr. Aesthetic Surg.* **2006**, *59*, 571–579. [CrossRef] [PubMed]
4. Santosa, K.B.; Qi, J.; Kim, H.M.; Hamill, J.B.; Wilkins, E.G.; Pusic, A.L. Long-Term Patient-Reported Outcomes in Postmastectomy Breast Reconstruction. *JAMA Surg.* **2018**, *153*, 891. [CrossRef] [PubMed]
5. Nelson, J.A.; Allen, R.J.; Polanco, T.; Shamsunder, M.; Patel, A.R.; McCarthy, C.M.; Matros, E.; Dayan, J.H.; Disa, J.J.; Cordeiro, P.G.; et al. Long-Term Patient-Reported Outcomes following Postmastectomy Breast Reconstruction: An 8-Year Examination of 3268 Patients. *Ann. Surg.* **2019**, *270*, 473–483. [CrossRef] [PubMed]
6. Miseré, R.M.; van Kuijk, S.M.; Claassens, E.L.; Heuts, E.M.; Piatkowski, A.A.; van der Hulst, R.R. Breast-Related and Body-Related Quality of Life Following Autologous Breast Reconstruction Is Superior to Implant-Based Breast Reconstruction—A Long-Term Follow-Up Study. *Breast* **2021**, *59*, 176–182. [CrossRef] [PubMed]
7. Messenger, D.; Carter, F.; Noble, E.; Francis, N. Electrosurgery and Energized Dissection. *Surgery* **2020**, *38*, 133–138. [CrossRef]
8. Loh, S.A.; Carlson, G.A.; Chang, E.I.; Huang, E.; Palanker, D.; Gurtner, G.C. Comparative Healing of Surgical Incisions Created by the PEAK Plasmablade, Conventional Electrosurgery, and a Scalpel. *Plast. Reconstr. Surg.* **2009**, *124*, 1849–1859. [CrossRef] [PubMed]
9. Palanker, D.V.; Vankov, A.; Huie, P. Electrosurgery with Cellular Precision. *IEEE Trans. Biomed. Eng.* **2008**, *55*, 838–841. [CrossRef]
10. Ruidiaz, M.E.; Messmer, D.; Atmodjo, D.Y.; Vose, J.G.; Huang, E.J.; Kummel, A.C.; Rosenberg, H.L.; Gurtner, G.C. Comparative Healing of Human Cutaneous Surgical Incisions Created by the PEAK PlasmaBlade, Conventional Electrosurgery, and a Standard Scalpel. *Plast. Reconstr. Surg.* **2011**, *128*, 104–111. [CrossRef]
11. Schlosshauer, T.; Kiehlmann, M.; Riener, M.O.; Rothenberger, J.; Sader, R.; Rieger, U.M. Effect of Low-Thermal Dissection Device versus Conventional Electrocautery in Mastectomy for Female-to-Male Transgender Patients. *Int. Wound J.* **2020**, *17*, 1239–1245. [CrossRef] [PubMed]
12. Xiao, X.; Ye, L. Efficacy and Safety of Scarpa Fascia Preservation during Abdominoplasty: A Systematic Review and Meta-Analysis. *Aesthetic Plast. Surg.* **2017**, *41*, 585–590. [CrossRef] [PubMed]
13. Wormald, J.C.R.; Wade, R.G.; Figus, A. The Increased Risk of Adverse Outcomes in Bilateral Deep Inferior Epigastric Artery Perforator Flap Breast Reconstruction Compared to Unilateral Reconstruction: A Systematic Review and Meta-Analysis. *J. Plast. Reconstr. Aesthetic Surg.* **2014**, *67*, 143–156. [CrossRef] [PubMed]

14. Salgarello, M.; Tambasco, D.; Farallo, E. DIEP Flap Donor Site Versus Elective Abdominoplasty Short-Term Complication Rates: A Meta-Analysis. *Aesthetic Plast. Surg.* **2012**, *36*, 363–369. [CrossRef] [PubMed]
15. Tan, M.Y.L.; Onggo, J.; Serag, S.; Phan, K.; Dusseldorp, J.R. Deep Inferior Epigastric Perforator (DIEP) Flap Safety Profile in Slim versus Non-Slim BMI Patients: A Systematic Review and Meta-Analysis. *J. Plast. Reconstr. Aesthet. Surg.* **2022**, *75*, 2180–2189. [CrossRef] [PubMed]
16. Mani, M.; Wang, T.; Harris, P.; James, S. Breast Reconstruction with the Deep Inferior Epigastric Perforator Flap is a Reliable Alternative In Slim Patients. *Microsurgery* **2016**, *36*, 552–558. [CrossRef] [PubMed]
17. Schlosshauer, T.; Kiehlmann, M.; Rothenberger, J.; Sader, R.; Rieger, U.M. Bilateral Reduction Mammaplasty with Pulsed Electron Avalanche Knife Plasmablade™ and Conventional Electrosurgical Surgery: A Retrospective, Randomised Controlled Clinical Trial. *Int. Wound J.* **2020**, *17*, 1695–1701. [CrossRef]
18. Schlosshauer, T.; Kiehlmann, M.; Riener, M.O.; Sader, R.; Rieger, U.M. Comparative Analysis on the Effect of Low-Thermal Plasma Dissection Device (PEAK PlasmaBlade) vs. Conventional Electrosurgery in Post-Bariatric Abdominoplasty: A Retrospective Randomised Clinical Study. *Int. Wound J.* **2019**, *16*, 1494–1502. [CrossRef]
19. Sowa, Y.; Inafuku, N.; Kodama, T.; Morita, D.; Numajiri, T. Preventive Effect on Seroma of Use of Peak Plasmablade after Latissimus Dorsi Breast Reconstruction. *Plast. Reconstr. Surg. Glob. Open* **2018**, *6*, e2035. [CrossRef] [PubMed]
20. Dogan, L.; Gulcelik, M.A.; Yuksel, M.; Uyar, O.; Erdogan, O.; Reis, E. The Effect of Plasmakinetic Cautery on Wound Healing and Complications in Mastectomy. *J. Breast Cancer* **2013**, *16*, 198–201. [CrossRef]
21. Friebel, T.R.; Narayan, N.; Ramakrishnan, V.; Morgan, M.; Cellek, S.; Griffiths, M. Comparison of PEAK PlasmaBlade™ to Conventional Diathermy in Abdominal-Based Free-Flap Breast Reconstruction Surgery—A Single-Centre Double-Blinded Randomised Controlled Trial. *J. Plast. Reconstr. Aesthet. Surg.* **2021**, *74*, 1731–1742. [CrossRef] [PubMed]
22. Chiappa, C.; Fachinetti, A.; Boeri, C.; Arlant, V.; Rausei, S.; Dionigi, G.; Rovera, F. Wound Healing and Postsurgical Complications in Breast Cancer Surgery: A Comparison between PEAK PlasmaBlade and Conventional Electrosurgery—A Preliminary Report of a Case Series. *Ann. Surg. Treat. Res.* **2018**, *95*, 129–134. [CrossRef]
23. Clavien, P.A.; Barkun, J.; De Oliveira, M.L.; Vauthey, J.N.; Dindo, D.; Schulick, R.D.; De Santibañes, E.; Pekolj, J.; Slankamenac, K.; Bassi, C.; et al. The Clavien-Dindo Classification of Surgical Complications: Five-Year Experience. *Ann. Surg.* **2009**, *250*, 187–196. [CrossRef]
24. Yilmaz, K.B.; Dogan, L.; Nalbant, H.; Akinci, M.; Karaman, N.; Ozaslan, C.; Kulacoglu, H. Comparing Scalpel, Electrocautery and Ultrasonic Dissector Effects: The Impact on Wound Complications And Pro-Inflammatory Cytokine Levels in Wound Fluid from Mastectomy Patients. *J. Breast Cancer* **2011**, *14*, 58. [CrossRef]
25. Duscher, D.; Aitzetmüller, M.M.; Shan, J.J.; Wenny, R.; Brett, E.A.; Staud, C.J.; Kiesl, D.; Huemer, G.M. Comparison of Energy-Based Tissue Dissection Techniques in Abdominoplasty: A Randomized, Open-Label Study Including Economic Aspects. *Aesthetic Surg. J.* **2019**, *39*, 536–543. [CrossRef] [PubMed]
26. Chow, W.T.H.; Oni, G.; Ramakrishnan, V.V.; Griffiths, M. The Use of Plasmakinetic Cautery Compared to Conventional Electrocautery for Dissection of Abdominal Free Flap for Breast Reconstruction: Single-Centre, Randomized Controlled Study. *Gland Surg.* **2019**, *8*, 242–248. [CrossRef]
27. Chen, A.W.G.; Chen, M.K. Comparison of Post-Tonsillectomy Hemorrhage between Monopolar and Plasma Blade Techniques. *J. Clin. Med.* **2021**, *10*, 2051. [CrossRef] [PubMed]
28. Lane, J.C.; Dworkin-Valenti, J.; Chiodo, L.; Haupert, M. Postoperative Tonsillectomy Bleeding Complications in Children: A Comparison of Three Surgical Techniques. *Int. J. Pediatr. Otorhinolaryngol.* **2016**, *88*, 184–188. [CrossRef] [PubMed]
29. Thottam, P.J.; Christenson, J.R.; Cohen, D.S.; Metz, C.M.; Saraiya, S.S.; Haupert, M.S. The Utility of Common Surgical Instruments for Pediatric Adenotonsillectomy. *Laryngoscope* **2015**, *125*, 475–479. [CrossRef] [PubMed]
30. Kypta, A.; Blessberger, H.; Saleh, K.; Hönig, S.; Kammler, J.; Neeser, K.; Steinwender, C. An Electrical Plasma Surgery Tool for Device Replacement—Retrospective Evaluation of Complications and Economic Evaluation of Costs and Resource Use. *Pacing Clin. Electrophysiol.* **2015**, *38*, 28–34. [CrossRef]
31. Decker, M.R.; Greenblatt, D.Y.; Havlena, J.; Wilke, L.G.; Greenberg, C.C.; Neuman, H.B. Impact of Neoadjuvant Chemotherapy on Wound Complications after Breast Surgery. *Surgery* **2012**, *152*, 382–388. [CrossRef] [PubMed]
32. Azzawi, K.; Ismail, A.; Earl, H.; Forouhi, P.; Malata, C.M. Influence of Neoadjuvant Chemotherapy on Outcomes of Immediate Breast Reconstruction. *Plast. Reconstr. Surg.* **2010**, *126*, 22. [CrossRef] [PubMed]
33. Bowen, M.E.; Mone, M.C.; Buys, S.S.; Sheng, X.; Nelson, E.W. Surgical Outcomes for Mastectomy Patients Receiving Neoadjuvant Chemotherapy. *Ann. Surg.* **2017**, *265*, 448–456. [CrossRef] [PubMed]
34. Varghese, J.; Gohari, S.S.; Rizki, H.; Faheem, I.; Langridge, B.; Kümmel, S.; Johnson, L.; Schmid, P. A Systematic Review and Meta-Analysis on the Effect of Neoadjuvant Chemotherapy on Complications Following Immediate Breast Reconstruction. *Breast* **2021**, *55*, 55–62. [CrossRef] [PubMed]
35. Song, J.; Zhang, X.; Liu, Q.; Peng, J.; Liang, X.; Shen, Y.; Liu, H.; Li, H. Impact of Neoadjuvant Chemotherapy on Immediate Breast Reconstruction: A Meta-Analysis. *PLoS ONE* **2014**, *9*, e98225. [CrossRef] [PubMed]
36. Heidekrueger, P.I.; Fritschen, U.; Moellhoff, N.; Germann, G.; Giunta, R.E.; Zeman, F.; Prantl, L. Impact of Body Mass Index on Free DIEP Flap Breast Reconstruction: A Multicenter Cohort Study. *J. Plast. Reconstr. Aesthet. Surg.* **2021**, *74*, 1718–1724. [CrossRef] [PubMed]

37. Kearns, S.R.; Connolly, E.M.; Mcnally, S.; Mcnamara, D.A.; Deasy, J. Randomized Clinical Trial of Diathermy versus Scalpel Incision in Elective Midline Laparotomy. *Br. J. Surg.* **2000**, *88*, 41–44. [CrossRef]
38. Chrysos, E.; Athanasakis, E.; Antonakakis, S.; Zoras, O. A Prospective Study Comparing Diathermy and Scalpel Incisions in Tension-Free Inguinal Hernioplasty. *Am. Surg.* **2005**, *71*, 326–329. [CrossRef]

Disclaimer/Publisher's Note: The statements, opinions and data contained in all publications are solely those of the individual author(s) and contributor(s) and not of MDPI and/or the editor(s). MDPI and/or the editor(s) disclaim responsibility for any injury to people or property resulting from any ideas, methods, instructions or products referred to in the content.

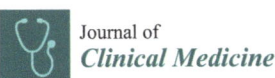

Article

High-Volume Liposuction in Lipedema Patients: Effects on Serum Vitamin D

Tonatiuh Flores [1,2,*], Celina Kerschbaumer [1], Florian J. Jaklin [3], Christina Glisic [1,2], Hugo Sabitzer [1,2], Jakob Nedomansky [1,2], Peter Wolf [4], Michael Weber [1], Konstantin D. Bergmeister [1,2,3] and Klaus F. Schrögendorfer [1,2]

[1] Karl Landsteiner University of Health Sciences, Dr. Karl-Dorrek-Straße 30, 3500 Krems, Austria; 51807592@edu.kl.ac.at (C.K.); christina.glisisc@stpoelten.lknoe.at (C.G.); hugo.sabitzer@stpoelten.lknoe.at (H.S.); jakob.nedomansky@stpoelten.lknoe.at (J.N.); michael.weber@kl.ac.at (M.W.); konstantin.bergmeister@stpoelten.lknoe.at (K.D.B.); klaus.schroegendorfer@stpoelten.lknoe.at (K.F.S.)
[2] Clinical Department of Plastic, Aesthetic and Reconstructive Surgery, University Clinic of St. Poelten, 3100 St. Poelten, Austria
[3] Clinical Laboratory for Bionic Extremity Reconstruction, University Clinic for Plastic, Reconstructive and Aesthetic Surgery, Medical University of Vienna, 1090 Vienna, Austria; florian.jaklin@meduniwien.ac.at
[4] Division of Endocrinology and Metabolism, Department of Internal Medicine III, Medical University of Vienna, 1090 Vienna, Austria; peter.wolf@meduniwien.ac.at
* Correspondence: t.flores@gmx.net; Tel.: +43-2742-9004-23624

Abstract: Background: Lipedema is a subcutaneous adipose tissue disorder characterized by increased pathological adipocytes mainly in the extremities. Vitamin D is stored in adipocytes, and serum levels inversely correlate with BMI. As adipocytes are removed during liposuction, lipedema patients might be prone to further substantial vitamin D loss while their levels are already decreased. Therefore, we examined the effect of liposuction on perioperative serum 25-hydroxyvitamin D levels. **Methods**: In patients undergoing lipedema liposuction, blood samples were obtained pre- and postoperatively. Statistical analyses were performed to correlate the volume of lipoaspirate, patients' BMI and number of sessions to vitamin D levels. **Results**: Overall, 213 patients were analyzed. Mean liposuction volume was 6615.33 ± 3884.25 mL, mean BMI was 32.18 ± 7.26 kg/m^2. mean preoperative vitamin D levels were 30.1 ± 14.45 ng/mL (borderline deficient according to the endocrine society) and mean postoperative vitamin D levels were 21.91 ± 9.18 ng/mL (deficient). A significant decrease in serum vitamin D was seen in our patients ($p < 0.001$) of mean 7.83 ng/mL. The amount of vitamin D loss was not associated with BMI or aspiration volume in our patients ($p > 0.05$). Interestingly, vitamin D dynamics showed a steady drop regardless of volume aspirated or preoperative levels. **Conclusions**: Many lipedema patients have low vitamin D levels preoperatively. Liposuction significantly reduced these levels additionally, regardless of aspirated volume or BMI. However, vitamin D loss was constant and predictable; thus, patients at risk are easily identified. Overall, lipedema patients undergoing liposuction are prone to vitamin D deficiency, and the long-term effects in this population are currently unknown.

Keywords: liposuction; lipedema; vitamin D; BMI

1. Introduction

Lipedema is a subcutaneous adipose tissue disorder almost solely affecting women [1,2]. Patients mainly suffer from painful localized fat deposition in the extremities with consecutive restrictions in daily life [2–4]. Due to its complex etiology and variable clinical manifestations, it presents as a multifaceted challenge for modern surgery. A vast number of comorbidities are associated with lipedema, such as hypertension, depression or increased BMI [5,6]. Vitamin D is stored in fat tissue, and due to its inverse correlation with

BMI status and body fat, vitamin D serum deficiency can frequently be seen in lipedema patients [5,7–16]. It is the most common deficiency in obese patients worldwide with a prevalence of 80–90% [9,17–25].

Besides their painful nature, lipedematous adipocytes are resistant to diets and bariatric surgery [6,26,27]. Despite growing recognition, effective treatment modalities for lipedema remain limited. Therefore, liposuction has emerged as the only suitable procedure for managing lipedema-related symptoms, offering symptomatic relief to reduce patients' burden and enhance their quality of life [25,26].

To our knowledge, this is the first study investigating the relationship of liposuction and vitamin D serum levels in lipedema patients. Hence, in this study we seek to critically examine the implications of vitamin D deficiency in lipedema patients after liposuction, elucidating the potential challenges and proposing strategies for mitigating adverse outcomes. We aimed to analyze perioperative vitamin D alternations in lipedema patients undergoing liposuction.

2. Materials and Methods

2.1. Study Design and Patient Analysis

In this study we analyzed pre- and postoperative vitamin D serum levels in lipedema patients undergoing liposuction at the Clinical Department for Plastic, Aesthetic and Reconstructive Surgery at the University Hospital St. Poelten, between 1 January 2018 and 31 December 2022. The study was conducted as a retrospective single center study. Ethical approval was obtained from the local institutional review board at the Karl Landsteiner University of Health Sciences Krems (reference number: ECS 1041/2021). Analyzed factors included the patients' age at surgery, BMI, volume of lipoaspiration, pre- and postoperative serum vitamin D levels, localization of treated area (upper and lower extremities) and liposuction sessions (one, two or three sessions).

2.2. Operative Procedure

At our department, liposuction is performed under general anesthesia using tumescent technique. Patients are examined and marked preoperatively while standing to assess areas to be treated. All patients receive intravenous antibiotic shielding with either 2.2 g of amoxicillin/clavulanic acid combination (Curam®, Sandoz GmbH, 6250 Kundl, Austria) or 600 mg of clindamycin (Dalacin®, Fareva Amboise Zone Industrielle, Routes des Industries 29, 37530 Pocé-sur-Cisse, France) in case of penicillin allergy. Antibiotic administration is given 30 min before surgical incision and is continued for one week postoperatively. Patients receive a modified Klein's solution with 1.000 mL Ringer's lactate (Ringer lactate®, Fresenius Kabi, Rue du Rempart 6, 27400 Louviers, France) containing 1 mL of 1:1.000 epinephrin (Suprarenin® Sanofi-Aventis GmbH, 65926 Frankfurt am Main, Germany). The solution is infiltrated with specialized infiltration cannulas through small stab incisions at strategically placed locations using a number 11 blade, which can easily be camouflaged postoperatively by the patient's clothing (e.g., the groin). After an indwelling time of approximately 15 min for the tumescent solution to set, vibration-assisted liposuction (VAL) is performed using Moeller's liposuction device (Moeller Vibrasat Pro, Moeller medical® GmbH, Wasserkuppenstraße 29-31, 36043 Fulda, Germany) with 3 and/or 4 mm multiport cannulas (multiport rapid extraction cannula, Moeller Medical® GmbH, Wasserkuppenstraße 29-31, 36043 Fulda, Germany) (Figure 1). Incisions are not sutured and are solely covered with plasters after antiseptic irrigation with Octenisept® (Schülke & Mayr GmbH, Robert-Koch-Straße 2, 22851, Norderstedt, Germany) and Skinsept® (Ecolab Germany GmbH, Ecolab-Allee 1, 40789 Monheim am Rhein, Germany). Compression garments are installed immediately postoperatively in the operating room. Compression garments are worn day and night for three months postoperatively. Patients receive antithrombotic shielding using low molecular heparin for 10 to 30 days postoperatively.

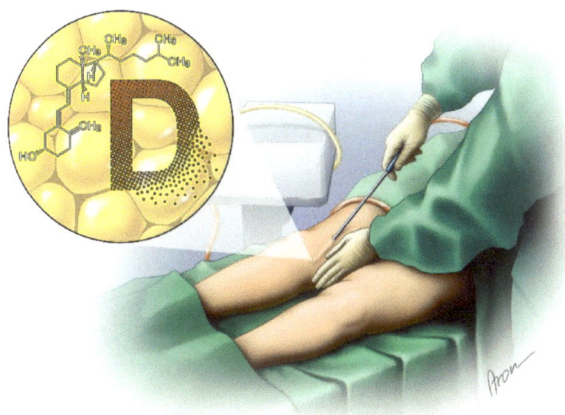

Figure 1. Illustration demonstrating the depletion of vitamin D during liposuction.

2.3. Blood Sampling

Blood samples were collected preoperatively at a maximum of one week prior to surgery and analyzed for serum 25-hydroxyvitamin D levels at our clinical institute of laboratory medicine. The vacutainers used for vitamin D sampling were BD Vacutainer® with stabilizing gel (Fischer Scientific GmbH, Im Heiligen Feld 17, 58239 Schwerte, Germany). Vitamin D components were separated using Elecsys Vitamin D total III Cobas® (Roche Diagnostics GmbH, Sandhofer Straße 116, 68305 Mannheim, Germany). All samples were retrieved and processed using the same instruments. Sample results were digitally stored at the hospital's data working space adhering to Austrian regulations for data protection. Postoperative sample collection was performed on the first postoperative day. Serum vitamin D levels below 30 ng/mL, according to the Endocrine Society were indicated as deficiency [28].

2.4. Statistics and Data Management

The endpoint of our analyses was to assess the alteration of vitamin D serum levels after liposuction and high-volume liposuction in lipedema patients. All data were reported anonymously. Data protection management complied with Austrian legislation. Data collection and processing were performed with Microsoft Excel (Software Version 2021, Microsoft Corp., One Microsoft Way, Redmond, 98052 Washington, DC, USA), and statistical analyses were performed using IBM SPSS Statistics version 26 (©IBM, Armonk, NY, USA). Nominal data were described using absolute frequencies and percentages. For metric data, mean and standard deviation were indicated. To correlate the volume of lipoaspirate and patients' BMI to vitamin D alterations, correlation analyses using Spearman's rho test were performed. Further, paired *t*-test analyses were conducted. Two-sided $p \leq 0.05$ was regarded as statistically significant. To analyze the decrease in vitamin D levels regarding liposuction sessions, analysis of variance (ANOVA) was used.

3. Results

3.1. Demographics

In total, 213 liposuctions in 100 patients suffering from lipedema were identified during the study period. Thereof, 163 liposuctions in 61 patients were excluded due to missing data (Figure 2).

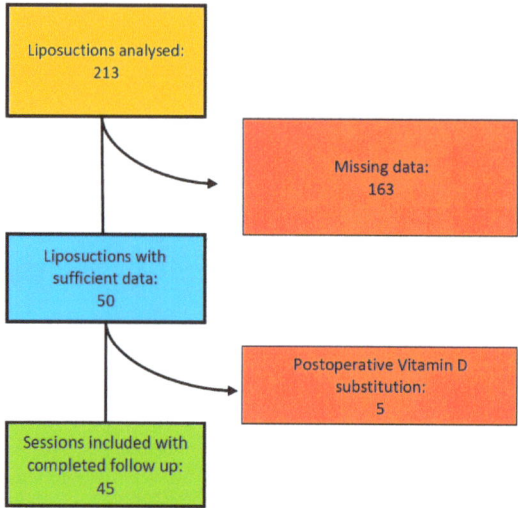

Figure 2. Organigram of patient selection for study inclusion.

Additionally, five liposuctions in three patients were excluded because of self-supplied postoperative vitamin D substitution. Consequently, 45 liposuctions in 36 patients met our criteria and were included in our study. We analyzed 35 liposuctions on lower extremities and 10 liposuctions on upper extremities (Figure 3). All patients included were Caucasian women and did not expose themselves excessively to the sun or substitute vitamin D independently according to the anamnesis.

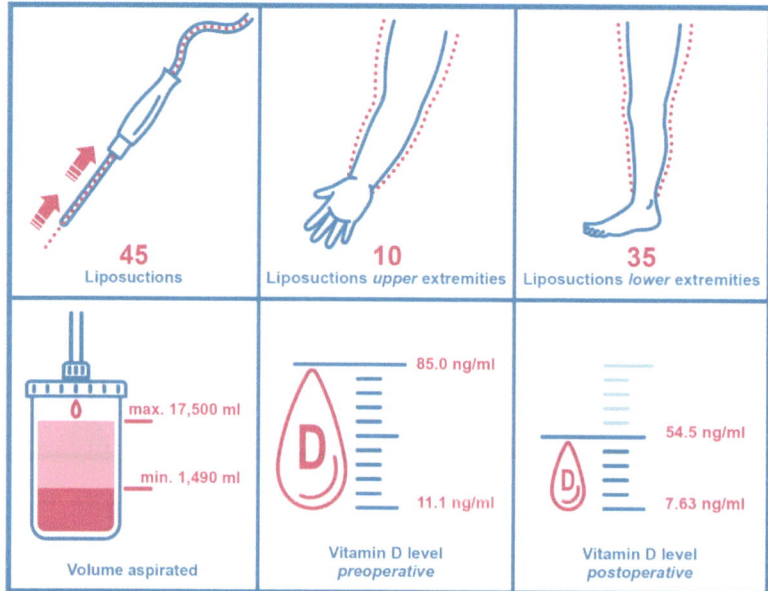

Figure 3. Key data chart of included study patients and clinical findings. Arrows and dotted lines in the upper left window show the suction path (arrows) of lipoaspirate (dotted lines) during liposuction.

Mean patient age was 38.11 ± 13.74 years overall, ranging from 19 years as the youngest to 71 years as the oldest at time of surgery (Table 1). Mean BMI was 32.18 ± 7.26 kg/m^2, varying from 21.7 kg/m^2 to 53.1 kg/m^2 (Table 1). Mean volume aspirated was 6615.33 ± 3884.253 mL, with a minimum of 1490 mL and maximum of 17,500 mL in one session (Table 1). Patients were further divided into two groups as higher volumes of liposuction mainly occur in the lower extremities: patients undergoing liposuction on upper extremities and patients undergoing liposuction on lower extremities.

Table 1. Baseline characteristics of patients. Significantly lower vitamin D serum levels can be observed postoperatively.

Patient Characteristics	Total	Upper Extremities	Lower Extremities
Number	45	10	35
Age—years mean (standard deviation)	38.11 (std.: 13.74)	39.0 (std.: 15.74)	37.86 (std.: 13.36)
min.–max.	19–71	20–57	19–71
BMI—kg/m^2 mean (standard deviation)	32.18 (std.: 7.26)	29.210 (std.: 3.96)	33.029 (std.: 7.79)
min.–max.	21.7–53.1	24.2–36.4	21.7–53.1
Vit D pre—ng/mL mean (standard deviation)	30.1 (std.: 14.45)	33.240 (std.: 14.66)	29.203 (std.: 14.47)
min.–max.	11.1–85.0	15.8–64.3	11.1–85.0
Vit D post—ng/mL mean (standard deviation)	21.914 (std.: 9.18)	25.85 (std.: 12.44)	20.7903 (std.: 7.89)
min.–max.	7.63–54.5	13.7–54.5	7.63–42.5
Volume—mL mean (standard deviation)	6615.33 (std.: 3884.25)	3.845 (std.: 3884.25)	7406.86 (std.: 3997.91)
min.–max.	1490–17,500	1800–7600	1490–17,500

3.2. Liposuction of Upper Extremities

Patients' mean age in this group was 39.0 ± 15.74 years, ranging from 20 years to 57 years. Mean BMI in the upper extremity group was 29.21 ± 3.96 kg/m^2, ranging from 24.2 kg/m^2 to 36.4 kg/m^2. Mean volume aspirated was 3845 mL ± 3884.25 mL with a minimum of 1800 mL and a maximum of 7600 mL in one session (Table 1).

3.3. Liposuction of Lower Extremities

In the lower extremity group, patients' mean age was 37.86 ± 13.36, ranging from 19 to 71 years. Mean BMI was 33.03 ± 7.79 kg/m^2, ranging from 21.7 kg/m^2 to 53.1 kg/m^2. Mean volume aspirated was 7406.86 ± 3997.92 mL with a minimum of 1490 mL and a maximum of 17,500 mL in one session (Table 1).

3.4. Vitamin D Serum Levels

In total, mean preoperative vitamin D levels were 30.1 ± 14.45 ng/mL, ranging from 11.1 ng/mL to 85.0 ng/mL (Table 1, Figure 4).

Mean postoperative vitamin D levels were 21.91 ± 9.18 ng/mL, ranging from 7.63 ng/mL to 54.5 ng/mL (Table 1, Figure 5).

In total, 29 patients showed preoperative vitamin D levels below 30 ng/mL. Postoperatively, 40 patients showed vitamin D levels below 30 ng/mL. None of our patients with preoperative vitamin D levels below 30 ng/mL showed any clinical sign of deficiencies. Vitamin D was not substituted in our cohort, either pre- or postoperatively.

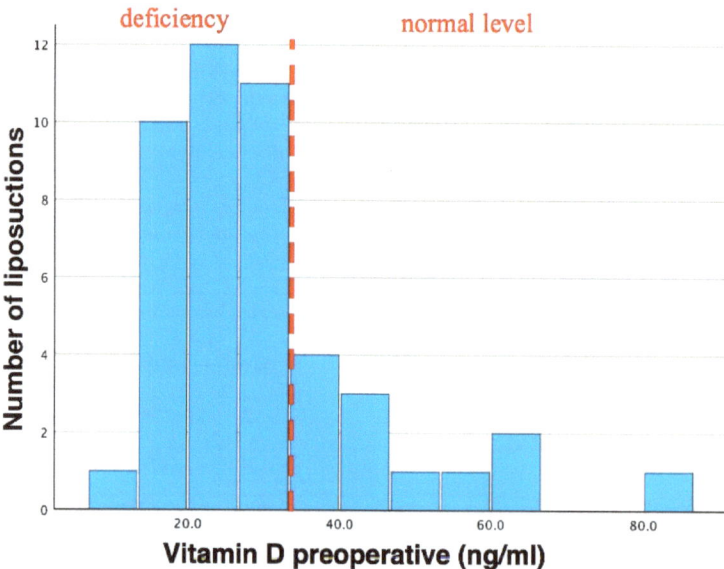

Figure 4. Histogram of preoperative vitamin D. Mean vitamin D levels were 30.1 ng/mL in total. Std. was 14.45 ng/mL (N = 46). Preoperative vitamin D insufficiency (according to the endocrine society) can be observed as most bars are shifted to the left. This vitamin D insufficiency is often seen in lipedema patients. Dotted line indicates the threshold of vitamin D deficiency to non-deficiency in preoperative patients.

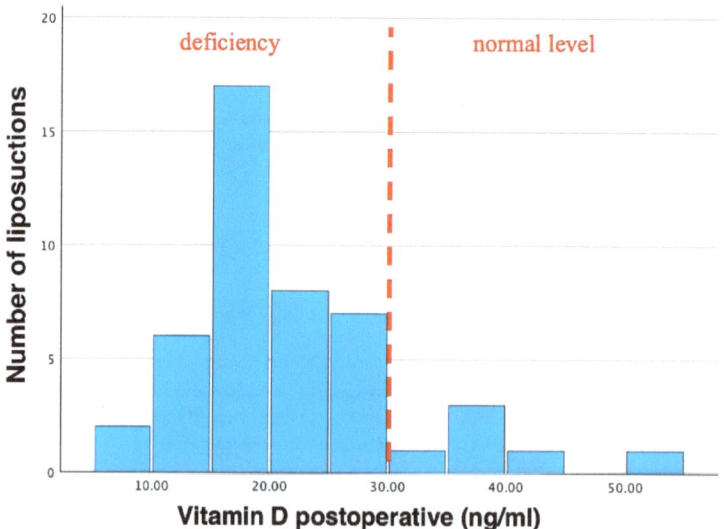

Figure 5. Histogram of postoperative vitamin D levels. Mean vitamin D was 21.91 ng/mL. Std. was 9.18 ng/mL (N = 46). A vitamin D insufficiency can clearly be seen in postoperative values as the bars are shifted to the left. Pre-existing vitamin D insufficiencies are further aggravated through liposuction. Dotted line indicates the threshold of vitamin D deficiency to non-deficiency in postoperative patients.

3.5. Vitamin D Serum Levels of Liposuction of Upper Extremities

In this group, mean preoperative vitamin D levels were 33.24 ± 14.66 ng/mL, displaying a range from 15.8 ng/mL to 64.3 ng/mL. Mean postoperative vitamin D levels were 25.85 ± 12.44 ng/mL, measuring from 13.7 ng/mL to 54.5 ng/mL (Table 1, Figure 3).

3.6. Vitamin D Serum Levels of Liposuction of Lower Extremities

Mean preoperative vitamin D levels were 29.20 ± 14.47 ng/mL, ranging from 11.1 ng/mL to 85.0 ng/mL in patients treated at lower extremities. Mean postoperative vitamin D levels were 20.79 ± 7.89 ng/mL, ranging from 7.63 ng/mL to 42.5 ng/mL (Table 1, Figure 3).

3.7. Correlation Analysis

We correlated patients' BMI with the amount of ml aspirated during liposuction, expecting a higher BMI drop at higher liposuction volumes. Using Spearman's rho test for rank correlation, our analyses showed no significant correlation, either in absolute numbers ($p = 0.006$) or in relative numbers ($p = 1.97$) (Table 2), demonstrating that the absolute amount of volume reduced does not interfere with the patients' BMI.

Table 2. Spearman's rho test for rank correlation demonstrating no significant correlation between the volume of fat removed and the decrease in patients' BMI (p-values > 0.05). Regardless of the volume aspirated, the difference in pre- and postoperative BMI did not show significant changes. This finding is displayed in absolute and relative numbers within this table.

Spearman's Rho			Volume Aspirated	BMI
		Spearman's Rho Correlation of Volume Aspirated and BMI		
	BMI	Correlation coefficient	0.632	
		Sig. (2-sided)	<0.001	
		N	45	
	Absolute decline	Correlation coefficient	0.006	0.052
		Sig. (2-sided)	0.969	0.732
		N	45	45
	Relative decline	Correlation coefficient	0.197	0.059
		Sig. (2-sided)	0.195	0.698
		N	45	45

Investigating the patients' vitamin D serum levels pre- and postoperatively, we found a statistically significant decrease regarding vitamin D levels using a paired t-test ($p < 0.001$, Table 3). These findings were both significant overall and between the different groups ($p < 0.001$, Table 3). Since our data set turned out not to be normally distributed (outliers included in our data set), we additionally conducted the according non-parametric tests. Nonetheless, our data were still significant, additionally supporting our statistical findings ($p < 0.001$; labeled in red, Table 3).

Table 3. t-Test analysis showing the significant correlation between the measured vitamin D serum levels pre- and postoperatively ($p < 0.001$).

		t-Test			
		Mean	N	Std.-Deviation	*p*-Value
Pairing	Vit. D pre	30.10	45	14.45	<0.001 / <0.001
	Vit. D post	21.91	45	9.18	

This demonstrates that high-volume liposuction has a significant impact on postoperative vitamin D level changes. The abovementioned findings were also significant when analyzing areas treated separately (upper extremities and lower extremities). Hence, the decrease in vitamin D after liposuction was significant, no matter of liposuction location ($p < 0.001$).

The abovementioned findings were also significant when analyzing areas treated separately (upper extremities and lower extremities, Table 4). Hence, the decrease in vitamin D after liposuction was significant, no matter the area treated ($p < 0.001$, Table 4). Again, p-values of non-perimetric tests for non-normal distribution were also significant ($p = 0.005$ in upper extremities and $p < 0.001$ in lower extremities; labeled in red, Table 4).

Table 4. *t*-Test analysis on account of vitamin D decrease after liposuction in upper and lower extremities, demonstrating the statistical significance $p < 0.001$ in both groups (arms and legs). *p*-Values were still significant after non-perimetric testing ($p < 0.001$ and $p = 0.005$; labeled in red).

		t-Test				
	Localization	Mean	N	Std. Deviation	*p*-Value	
Legs	Vit. D pre	29.203	35	14.4755	<0.001/<0.001	
	Vit. D post	20.7903	35	7.89464		
Arms	Vit. D pre	33.240	10	14.6677	<0.001/0.005	
	Vit. D post	25.8500	10	12.44412		

Interestingly, after performing ANOVA (analysis of variance) for correlation of vitamin D level changes and the volume aspirated, we did not find any significant correlation ($p = 0.906$ in absolute numbers, and $p = 0.451$ in relative numbers, Table 5). This finding was also seen in non-perimetric testing ($p = 0.481$ in absolute numbers, and $p = 0.128$ in relative numbers; labeled in red, Table 5). These findings were consistent throughout the session of liposuction.

Table 5. Analysis of variance (ANOVA) of volume aspirated during liposuction and decrease in serum vitamin D levels. Here, no significant correlation can be observed ($p = 0.906$ in absolute numbers, and $p = 0.451$ in relative numbers), More likely, our ANOVA analysis shows a non-correlation, concluding that no matter the amount of volume aspirated, vitamin D levels do not drop concordantly. Rather, a stable decrease in vitamin D can be seen regardless of volume of lipoaspirate.

						95% Mean Confidence Interval	
		N	Mean	Std. Deviation	*p*-Value	Lower Limit	Upper Limit
Absolute decrease	1	22	8.81	13.16	0.906/0.481	2.98	14.65
	2	20	7.68	3.58		6.00	9.36
	3	3	6.86	8.01		−13.04	26.77
	total	45	8.18	9.57		5.30	11.06
Relative decrease	1	22	23.03	17.35	0.451/0.128	15.34	30.73
	2	20	27.19	10.53		22.26	32.12
	3	3	17.57	11.76		−11.64	46.80
	total	45	24.52	14.33		20.21	28.83

The findings demonstrate that no matter the volume removed during liposuction, vitamin D levels did not drop concordantly. Our analyses rather showed a non-correlation between the decrease in vitamin D after liposuction and the volume aspirated, hence demonstrating a stable drop in vitamin D between a mean of 6.86 ng/mL and 8.81 ng/mL (mean 7.83 ng/mL) no matter the volume of lipoaspirate.

4. Discussion

Many studies have been conducted to analyze serum levels of vitamin D after diets or bariatric surgery [10–12,29–33], yet none have investigated the alteration in vitamin D levels after liposuction in lipedema patients. To our knowledge, this is the first study investigating the correlation of vitamin D serum levels after liposuction.

Adipose tissue plays a significant role in energy supply and distribution and is essential in storing fat-soluble vitamins, such as vitamin D. Its bioactivity includes the reduction in inflammatory processes, neuromuscular regulation as well as the absorption of calcium, an essential mineral in osteosynthesis [29,34]. Vitamin D deficiency can lead to diminished immune responses, muscle weakness, osteoporosis and increased fracture rates [19,22,23,34–37]. Approximately 1 billion people (developing and developed countries) suffer from vitamin D deficiency, consequently making it a global public health issue [20,21,37,38]. It is the most common deficiency in obese patients worldwide [9,17–25]. Vitamin D is normally synthesized through the skin, yet obese patients have significantly lower levels in their blood stream compared to non-obese patients, despite having increased body surfaces [8,19,39]. This results from the inverse correlation of vitamin D and the patients' BMI, as more adipocytes store more vitamin D [5,7–15], thus, leading to serum deficiency. Since most lipedema patients have elevated BMI due to pathologically engorged adipocyte, this cohort often shows vitamin D deficiency as well. These patients not only display low vitamin D serum levels due to its inverse correlation to BMI but also because engorged and inflamed adipocytes in lipedema traps vitamin D [14,40–42]. This bidirectional relationship between vitamin D deficiency and elevated BMI with low serum vitamin D levels is also evident in our study.

Several studies have demonstrated that weight loss by lifestyle changes or bariatric surgeries increases vitamin D levels [8,10,11,29,43,44]. Nevertheless, this effect was not detected in our study after liposuction so far. Contrarily, our results showed a significant decrease in postoperative vitamin D levels after treatment (Figure 5).

Since liposuction is the gold standard in treating lipedema, patients already suffering from vitamin D deficiency are at risk of further vitamin D loss. The lack of vitamin D has already been linked to entailing chronic cellular stress, which can be seen in lipedema patients [40,42,45]. By further diminishing vitamin D levels after liposuction, patients experiencing lipedema further maintain oxidative stress, resulting in sustained lipedema symptoms [14,42,45]. Thus, lipedema symptoms might not ameliorate after treatment, potentially aggravating their symptoms. Although the postoperative 25-hydroxyvitamin D decrease did not drop concordantly with the volume aspirated, its decrease was significant in our findings. Therefore, lipedema patients ought to be screened for vitamin D deficiency and, if needed, it should be substituted to prevent further sequelae, such as osteopenia or osteoporosis.

To personalize liposuction for lipedema patients, preoperative assessment of vitamin D levels in concordance with the estimated amount of lipoaspirate is needed. Thereby, vitamin D levels can be improved before surgery and ensure patients face the operation in an optimized manner. Parenthetically, high-volume liposuction needs to be separated into several sessions to obviate excessive vitamin D loss postoperatively. Vitamin D levels in addition are to be monitored precisely between sessions to prevent patients from experiencing vitamin D deficiency in between treatment sessions. Interdisciplinary collaboration involving endocrinologists and nutritionists is essential for implementing patient-tailored strategies. Perioperative optimization of nutrition management or the administration of supplements to individually address the needs of lipedema patients is therefore favored to guarantee long-term patient safety.

5. Conclusions

Although liposuction is a relatively safe procedure, its aftereffects are not to be neglected. To protect this patient cohort from further long-term sequelae and to sufficiently relieve patients' burden, perioperative improvement of treatment modalities is necessary. By addressing vitamin D deficiency comprehensively, healthcare providers can enhance the efficacy of liposuction as a therapeutic tool for managing lipedema. To reduce postoperative vitamin D loss in lipedema patients, high-volume liposuction ought to be stratified and personalized to each patient individually for optimized vitamin D preservation. Therefore, lipedema patients might not suffer further comorbidities related to their underlying disease after treatment. Despite the significant findings in our research, our study faces a few limitations. Postoperative vitamin D levels should be monitored over a longer period. Also, the storage behavior and characteristics of lipedema adipocytes ought to be investigated through controlled histological analyses. Additional cross-section studies are needed for further detection of this underacknowledged threat.

Author Contributions: Conceptualization, T.F., C.K., F.J.J., C.G., H.S., J.N., P.W., M.W., K.D.B. and K.F.S.; methodology, T.F., C.K., F.J.J., C.G., H.S., J.N., P.W., M.W., K.D.B. and K.F.S.; validation, T.F., C.K., F.J.J., C.G., H.S., J.N., P.W., M.W., K.D.B. and K.F.S.; formal analysis, T.F., C.K., F.J.J., C.G., H.S., J.N., P.W., M.W., K.D.B. and K.F.S.; investigation, T.F., C.K., F.J.J., C.G., H.S., J.N., P.W., M.W., K.D.B. and K.F.S.; resources, T.F., C.K., F.J.J., C.G., H.S., J.N., P.W., M.W., K.D.B. and K.F.S.; data curation, T.F., C.K., F.J.J., C.G., H.S., J.N., P.W., M.W., K.D.B. and K.F.S.; writing—original draft preparation, T.F., C.K., F.J.J., C.G., H.S., J.N., P.W., M.W., K.D.B. and K.F.S.; writing—review and editing, T.F., C.K., F.J.J., C.G., H.S., J.N., P.W., M.W., K.D.B. and K.F.S.; visualization, T.F., C.K., F.J.J., C.G., H.S., J.N., P.W., M.W., K.D.B. and K.F.S.; supervision, K.D.B. and K.F.S.; project administration, T.F.; funding acquisition, T.F. All authors have read and agreed to the published version of the manuscript.

Funding: This research received funding for open access publication by the Karl Landsteiner University of Health Sciences, Dr. Karl-Dorrek-Straße 30, 3500, Krems, Austria.

Institutional Review Board Statement: The study was conducted according to the guidelines of the Declaration of Helsinki and approved by the Institutional Ethics Committee of Karl Landsteiner University of Health Sciences Krems (protocol code: 1041/2021, 2 November 2021).

Informed Consent Statement: Patient consent was waived due to the retrospective character of this study.

Data Availability Statement: All the data analyzed during the current study are available from the corresponding author on reasonable request.

Acknowledgments: The authors want to show appreciation for the contribution of NÖ Landesgesundheitsagentur, the legal entity of University Hospitals in Lower Austria, for providing the organizational framework to conduct this research. The authors also would like to acknowledge support from the Open Access Publishing Fund of Karl Landsteiner University of Health Sciences, Krems, Austria. This work was supported by Forschungsimpulse [project ID: SF_56], a program of Karl Landsteiner University of Health Sciences, funded by the Federal Government of Lower Austria. We also thank Aron Cserveny for providing the graphics. Open Access Funding by Karl Landsteiner University of Health Sciences, Krems, Austria.

Conflicts of Interest: The authors declare no conflicts of interest.

References

1. Okhovat, J.P.; Alavi, A. Lipedema: A Review of the Literature. *Int. J. Low. Extrem. Wounds* **2015**, *14*, 262–267. [CrossRef] [PubMed]
2. Wollina, U. Lipedema-An update. *Dermatol. Ther.* **2019**, *32*, e12805. [CrossRef] [PubMed]
3. Katzer, K.; Hill, J.L.; McIver, K.B.; Foster, M.T. Lipedema and the Potential Role of Estrogen in Excessive Adipose Tissue Accumulation. *Int. J. Mol. Sci.* **2021**, *22*, 11720. [CrossRef] [PubMed]
4. Michelini, S.; Chiurazzi, P.; Marino, V.; Dell'Orco, D.; Manara, E.; Baglivo, M.; Fiorentino, A.; Maltese, P.E.; Pinelli, M.; Herbst, K.L.; et al. Aldo-Keto Reductase 1C1 (AKR1C1) as the First Mutated Gene in a Family with Nonsyndromic Primary Lipedema. *Int. J. Mol. Sci.* **2020**, *21*, 6264. [CrossRef] [PubMed]
5. Al-Wardat, M.; Alwardat, N.; Lou De Santis, G.; Zomparelli, S.; Gualtieri, P.; Bigioni, G.; Romano, L.; Di Renzo, L. The association between serum vitamin D and mood disorders in a cohort of lipedema patients. *Horm. Mol. Biol. Clin. Investig.* **2021**, *42*, 351–355. [CrossRef] [PubMed]
6. Bauer, A.T.; von Lukowicz, D.; Lossagk, K.; Aitzetmueller, M.; Moog, P.; Cerny, M.; Erne, H.; Schmauss, D.; Duscher, D.; Machens, H.G. New Insights on Lipedema: The Enigmatic Disease of the Peripheral Fat. *Plast. Reconstr. Surg.* **2019**, *144*, 1475–1484. [CrossRef]
7. Vranic, L.; Mikolasevic, I.; Milic, S. Vitamin D Deficiency: Consequence or Cause of Obesity? *Medicina* **2019**, *55*, 541. [CrossRef] [PubMed]
8. Walsh, J.S.; Bowles, S.; Evans, A.L. Vitamin D in obesity. *Curr. Opin. Endocrinol. Diabetes Obes.* **2017**, *24*, 389–394. [CrossRef] [PubMed]
9. Kobylinska, M.; Antosik, K.; Decyk, A.; Kurowska, K. Malnutrition in Obesity: Is It Possible? *Obes. Facts* **2022**, *15*, 19–25. [CrossRef] [PubMed]

10. Gangloff, A.; Bergeron, J.; Pelletier-Beaumont, E.; Nazare, J.A.; Smith, J.; Borel, A.L.; Lemieux, I.; Tremblay, A.; Poirier, P.; Almeras, N.; et al. Effect of adipose tissue volume loss on circulating 25-hydroxyvitamin D levels: Results from a 1-year lifestyle intervention in viscerally obese men. *Int. J. Obes.* **2015**, *39*, 1638–1643. [CrossRef]
11. Pramyothin, P.; Biancuzzo, R.M.; Lu, Z.; Hess, D.T.; Apovian, C.M.; Holick, M.F. Vitamin D in adipose tissue and serum 25-hydroxyvitamin D after roux-en-Y gastric bypass. *Obesity* **2011**, *19*, 2228–2234. [CrossRef] [PubMed]
12. Mallard, S.R.; Howe, A.S.; Houghton, L.A. Vitamin D status and weight loss: A systematic review and meta-analysis of randomized and nonrandomized controlled weight-loss trials. *Am. J. Clin. Nutr.* **2016**, *104*, 1151–1159. [CrossRef]
13. Carrelli, A.; Bucovsky, M.; Horst, R.; Cremers, S.; Zhang, C.; Bessler, M.; Schrope, B.; Evanko, J.; Blanco, J.; Silverberg, S.J.; et al. Vitamin D Storage in Adipose Tissue of Obese and Normal Weight Women. *J. Bone Miner. Res.* **2017**, *32*, 237–242. [CrossRef] [PubMed]
14. Bennour, I.; Haroun, N.; Sicard, F.; Mounien, L.; Landrier, J.F. Vitamin D and Obesity/Adiposity-A Brief Overview of Recent Studies. *Nutrients* **2022**, *14*, 2049. [CrossRef]
15. Borel, P.; Caillaud, D.; Cano, N.J. Vitamin D bioavailability: State of the art. *Crit. Rev. Food Sci. Nutr.* **2015**, *55*, 1193–1205. [CrossRef] [PubMed]
16. Herbst, K.L.; Kahn, L.A.; Iker, E.; Ehrlich, C.; Wright, T.; McHutchison, L.; Schwartz, J.; Sleigh, M.; Donahue, P.M.; Lisson, K.H.; et al. Standard of care for lipedema in the United States. *Phlebology* **2021**, *36*, 779–796. [CrossRef]
17. Via, M. The malnutrition of obesity: Micronutrient deficiencies that promote diabetes. *ISRN Endocrinol.* **2012**, *2012*, 103472. [CrossRef] [PubMed]
18. Guardiola-Marquez, C.E.; Santos-Ramirez, M.T.; Segura-Jimenez, M.E.; Figueroa-Montes, M.L.; Jacobo-Velazquez, D.A. Fighting Obesity-Related Micronutrient Deficiencies through Biofortification of Agri-Food Crops with Sustainable Fertilization Practices. *Plants* **2022**, *11*, 3477. [CrossRef]
19. Tobias, D.K.; Luttmann-Gibson, H.; Mora, S.; Danik, J.; Bubes, V.; Copeland, T.; LeBoff, M.S.; Cook, N.R.; Lee, I.M.; Buring, J.E.; et al. Association of Body Weight with Response to Vitamin D Supplementation and Metabolism. *JAMA Netw. Open* **2023**, *6*, e2250681. [CrossRef] [PubMed]
20. Nair, R.; Maseeh, A. Vitamin D: The "sunshine" vitamin. *J. Pharmacol. Pharmacother.* **2012**, *3*, 118–126.
21. Gordon, C.M.; DePeter, K.C.; Feldman, H.A.; Grace, E.; Emans, S.J. Prevalence of vitamin D deficiency among healthy adolescents. *Arch. Pediatr. Adolesc. Med.* **2004**, *158*, 531–537. [CrossRef] [PubMed]
22. Holick, M.F. The vitamin D deficiency pandemic: Approaches for diagnosis, treatment and prevention. *Rev. Endocr. Metab. Disord.* **2017**, *18*, 153–165. [CrossRef] [PubMed]
23. Holick, M.F.; Binkley, N.C.; Bischoff-Ferrari, H.A.; Gordon, C.M.; Hanley, D.A.; Heaney, R.P.; Murad, M.H.; Weaver, C.M.; Endocrine, S. Evaluation, treatment, and prevention of vitamin D deficiency: An Endocrine Society clinical practice guideline. *J. Clin. Endocrinol. Metab.* **2011**, *96*, 1911–1930. [CrossRef] [PubMed]
24. Bartley, J. Vitamin D: Emerging roles in infection and immunity. *Expert. Rev. Anti Infect. Ther.* **2010**, *8*, 1359–1369. [CrossRef] [PubMed]
25. Ghods, M.; Georgiou, I.; Schmidt, J.; Kruppa, P. Disease progression and comorbidities in lipedema patients: A 10-year retrospective analysis. *Dermatol. Ther.* **2020**, *33*, e14534. [CrossRef] [PubMed]
26. Dudek, J.E.; Bialaszek, W.; Ostaszewski, P. Quality of life in women with lipoedema: A contextual behavioral approach. *Qual. Life Res.* **2016**, *25*, 401–408. [CrossRef] [PubMed]
27. Fife, C.E.; Maus, E.A.; Carter, M.J. Lipedema: A frequently misdiagnosed and misunderstood fatty deposition syndrome. *Adv. Skin. Wound Care* **2010**, *23*, 81–92. [CrossRef] [PubMed]
28. Giustina, A.; Bilezikian, J.P.; Adler, R.A.; Banfi, G.; Bikle, D.D.; Binkley, N.C.; Bollerslev, J.; Bouillon, R.; Brandi, M.L.; Casanueva, F.F.; et al. Consensus Statement on Vitamin D Status Assessment and Supplementation: Whys, Whens, and Hows. *Endocr. Rev.* **2024**, bnae009. [CrossRef]
29. Buscemi, S.; Buscemi, C.; Corleo, D.; De Pergola, G.; Caldarella, R.; Meli, F.; Randazzo, C.; Milazzo, S.; Barile, A.M.; Rosafio, G.; et al. Obesity and Circulating Levels of Vitamin D before and after Weight Loss Induced by a Very Low-Calorie Ketogenic Diet. *Nutrients* **2021**, *13*, 1829. [CrossRef] [PubMed]
30. Lespessailles, E.; Toumi, H. Vitamin D alteration associated with obesity and bariatric surgery. *Exp. Biol. Med.* **2017**, *242*, 1086–1094. [CrossRef] [PubMed]
31. Goldner, W.S.; Stoner, J.A.; Lyden, E.; Thompson, J.; Taylor, K.; Larson, L.; Erickson, J.; McBride, C. Finding the optimal dose of vitamin D following Roux-en-Y gastric bypass: A prospective, randomized pilot clinical trial. *Obes. Surg.* **2009**, *19*, 173–179. [CrossRef] [PubMed]
32. Carlin, A.M.; Rao, D.S.; Yager, K.M.; Parikh, N.J.; Kapke, A. Treatment of vitamin D depletion after Roux-en-Y gastric bypass: A randomized prospective clinical trial. *Surg. Obes. Relat. Dis.* **2009**, *5*, 444–449. [CrossRef] [PubMed]
33. Chakhtoura, M.T.; Nakhoul, N.; Akl, E.A.; Mantzoros, C.S.; El Hajj Fuleihan, G.A. Guidelines on vitamin D replacement in bariatric surgery: Identification and systematic appraisal. *Metabolism* **2016**, *65*, 586–597. [CrossRef] [PubMed]
34. Bikle, D.D. Vitamin D metabolism, mechanism of action, and clinical applications. *Chem. Biol.* **2014**, *21*, 319–329. [CrossRef] [PubMed]
35. Schoenmakers, I.; Goldberg, G.R.; Prentice, A. Abundant sunshine and vitamin D deficiency. *Br. J. Nutr.* **2008**, *99*, 1171–1173. [CrossRef] [PubMed]

36. Reid, I.R.; Bolland, M.J.; Grey, A. Effects of vitamin D supplements on bone mineral density: A systematic review and meta-analysis. *Lancet* **2014**, *383*, 146–155. [CrossRef] [PubMed]
37. Heaney, R.P. Vitamin D in health and disease. *Clin. J. Am. Soc. Nephrol.* **2008**, *3*, 1535–1541. [CrossRef] [PubMed]
38. Lips, P.; Hosking, D.; Lippuner, K.; Norquist, J.M.; Wehren, L.; Maalouf, G.; Ragi-Eis, S.; Chandler, J. The prevalence of vitamin D inadequacy amongst women with osteoporosis: An international epidemiological investigation. *J. Intern. Med.* **2006**, *260*, 245–254. [CrossRef] [PubMed]
39. Parikh, S.J.; Edelman, M.; Uwaifo, G.I.; Freedman, R.J.; Semega-Janneh, M.; Reynolds, J.; Yanovski, J.A. The relationship between obesity and serum 1,25-dihydroxy vitamin D concentrations in healthy adults. *J. Clin. Endocrinol. Metab.* **2004**, *89*, 1196–1199. [CrossRef] [PubMed]
40. Poojari, A.; Dev, K.; Rabiee, A. Lipedema: Insights into Morphology, Pathophysiology, and Challenges. *Biomedicines* **2022**, *10*, 3081. [CrossRef] [PubMed]
41. Verde, L.; Camajani, E.; Annunziata, G.; Sojat, A.; Marina, L.V.; Colao, A.; Caprio, M.; Muscogiuri, G.; Barrea, L. Ketogenic Diet: A Nutritional Therapeutic Tool for Lipedema? *Curr. Obes. Rep.* **2023**, *12*, 529–543. [CrossRef] [PubMed]
42. Della Nera, G.; Sabatino, L.; Gaggini, M.; Gorini, F.; Vassalle, C. Vitamin D Determinants, Status, and Antioxidant/Anti-inflammatory-Related Effects in Cardiovascular Risk and Disease: Not the Last Word in the Controversy. *Antioxidants* **2023**, *12*, 948. [CrossRef] [PubMed]
43. Pereira-Santos, M.; Costa, P.R.; Assis, A.M.; Santos, C.A.; Santos, D.B. Obesity and vitamin D deficiency: A systematic review and meta-analysis. *Obes. Rev.* **2015**, *16*, 341–349. [CrossRef]
44. Drincic, A.T.; Armas, L.A.; Van Diest, E.E.; Heaney, R.P. Volumetric dilution, rather than sequestration best explains the low vitamin D status of obesity. *Obesity* **2012**, *20*, 1444–1448. [CrossRef] [PubMed]
45. Park, C.Y.; Han, S.N. The Role of Vitamin D in Adipose Tissue Biology: Adipocyte Differentiation, Energy Metabolism, and Inflammation. *J. Lipid Atheroscler.* **2021**, *10*, 130–144. [CrossRef] [PubMed]

Disclaimer/Publisher's Note: The statements, opinions and data contained in all publications are solely those of the individual author(s) and contributor(s) and not of MDPI and/or the editor(s). MDPI and/or the editor(s) disclaim responsibility for any injury to people or property resulting from any ideas, methods, instructions or products referred to in the content.

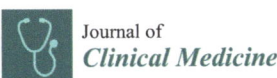

Article

Advancing Fingertip Regeneration: Outcomes from a New Conservative Treatment Protocol

Daihun Kang

Department of Plastic and Reconstructive Surgery, Ewha Womans University Seoul Hospital, Seoul 03760, Republic of Korea; gpk1234567@naver.com; Tel.: +82-10-4724-1419

Abstract: Background Fingertip injuries with volar pulp tissue defects present a significant challenge in management. This study aimed to evaluate the efficacy of a conservative treatment protocol using artificial dermis and semi-occlusive dressings for these injuries. **Methods** A single-center, prospective study was conducted on 31 patients with fingertip injuries involving volar pulp defects. The treatment protocol included wound debridement, application of artificial dermis (Pelnac®), and a semi-occlusive dressing (IV3000®). The outcomes were assessed using subjective questionnaires and objective measures, including fingerprint regeneration, sensory function, pain, and cosmetic appearance. **Results** The mean treatment duration was 45.29 days (SD = 17.53). Complications were minimal, with only one case (3.22%) directly attributable to the treatment. Fingerprint regeneration was considerable (mean score = 2.58, SD = 0.67). The sensory disturbances were minimal, with no significant differences across injury types. Post-treatment pain was low (mean = 0.45, SD = 0.67), and cosmetic satisfaction was high (mean = 4.09, SD = 0.94). The overall patient satisfaction was high (mean = 4.41, SD = 0.67), regardless of injury severity. **Conclusions** The conservative treatment protocol using artificial dermis and semi-occlusive dressings is a promising strategy for managing fingertip injuries with volar pulp defects. This approach minimizes surgical morbidity and achieves excellent functional and aesthetic outcomes.

Keywords: artificial dermis; fingertip; fingerprint; Pelnac®; reconstruction; regeneration; semi-occlusive; volar

1. Introduction

The human hand, a masterpiece of intricate anatomy and functional harmony, is our primary tool for exploring and interacting with the world around us. At the very tips of our fingers lies the volar pulp—a highly specialized structure essential for fine-touch sensation, grip stability, and precise manipulation [1,2]. This complex interplay of sensory and motor functions is made possible by the rich neurovascular network and specialized sensory receptors within the pulp [2]. However, the same complexity that endows the fingertips with their remarkable abilities also renders them particularly vulnerable to injury. Fingertip injuries involving volar pulp tissue defects can lead to significant functional impairment, sensory disturbances, and cosmetic disfigurement, ultimately impacting the patient's quality of life [3,4].

Traditionally, surgical approaches, such as local flaps, skin grafts, and free tissue transfers, have been employed to manage fingertip injuries with volar pulp defects [3,5–9]. While these techniques aim to restore the soft tissue envelope and preserve finger length, they are often associated with donor site morbidity, prolonged immobilization, and the need for multiple surgeries [3,4,10]. Moreover, these surgical interventions may not adequately restore the intricate sensory and biomechanical properties of the native pulp tissue, leading to suboptimal functional outcomes [4,11–13].

In pursuit of more effective and less invasive treatment options, there has been a growing interest in conservative approaches that harness the body's inherent regenerative potential [14]. The use of artificial dermal substitutes, such as Pelnac® (Gunze Limited, Kyoto, Japan), has shown promising results in managing various soft tissue defects [15–18]. These biomaterials provide a three-dimensional scaffold that mimics the natural extracellular matrix, facilitating cell migration, proliferation, and differentiation [19,20].

While previous studies have investigated the use of artificial dermis or semi-occlusive dressings separately in the treatment of fingertip injuries [18,21–24], the potential synergistic effects of combining these two approaches have not been extensively explored. Drawing inspiration from the adage that the whole is greater than the sum of its parts, this study aims to evaluate the efficacy of a novel conservative treatment protocol that combines the use of artificial dermis (Pelnac®) with a semi-occlusive dressing (IV3000®) in managing fingertip injuries with volar pulp tissue defects.

The rationale behind this combination is that the artificial dermis provides a structured scaffold for tissue regeneration, while the semi-occlusive dressing maintains a moist wound environment and allows for gas exchange [19,22,24,25]. The author hypothesizes that this synergistic approach will promote the regeneration of vascularized and innervated pulp tissue, leading to superior functional and aesthetic outcomes compared to traditional surgical interventions or conservative treatments using either artificial dermis or semi-occlusive dressings alone.

The potential benefits of this novel treatment protocol are multifaceted. First, it may reduce healing time and minimize complications associated with purely conservative treatments [20]. Second, it could lead to improved long-term functional and aesthetic outcomes by supporting the regeneration of complex tissue architecture [20,25,26]. Finally, despite the higher initial cost, this approach may prove to be cost-effective in the long run by achieving superior clinical outcomes and reducing the need for additional interventions [18].

To test this hypothesis and evaluate the effectiveness of this new combination protocol, a prospective study was conducted with the following primary objectives:

1. Assess the regeneration of volar pulp tissue, including the restoration of fingerprint pattern, sensory function, and cosmetic appearance.
2. Evaluate the impact of injury characteristics, such as bone or tendon exposure, on treatment outcomes and duration.
3. Investigate the incidence of complications and patient-reported outcomes, including pain, sensory disturbances, and overall satisfaction.
4. Compare the treatment duration and outcomes with those reported in previous studies utilizing artificial dermis or semi-occlusive dressings separately for fingertip reconstruction.

This study aims to provide valuable insights into the efficacy and feasibility of this novel treatment for managing fingertip injuries with volar pulp tissue defects.

2. Materials and Methods

A single-center, prospective study was conducted at our institution, which was approved by the Institutional Review Board (IRB) of the Catholic Kwandong University International St. Mary's Hospital (Approval No. 19 year IRB069, Registration No. IS19EISE0072). This study was performed in strict adherence to ethical guidelines. Written informed consent was obtained from all participants or their guardians prior to participation in this study. The study period was from December 2019 to December 2022, focusing on patients presenting with volar pulp tissue defects of the fingertip (Figure 1).

To ensure robust statistical power, a power analysis was conducted prior to patient recruitment. The analysis determined that a minimum of 30 patients in total was necessary to adequately power this study, assuming an alpha of 0.05, a power of 0.80, and an effect size of 0.5. This sample size was chosen to ensure that the study results would be statistically significant and replicable in similar clinical settings. Written informed consent was obtained from all participants involved in this study.

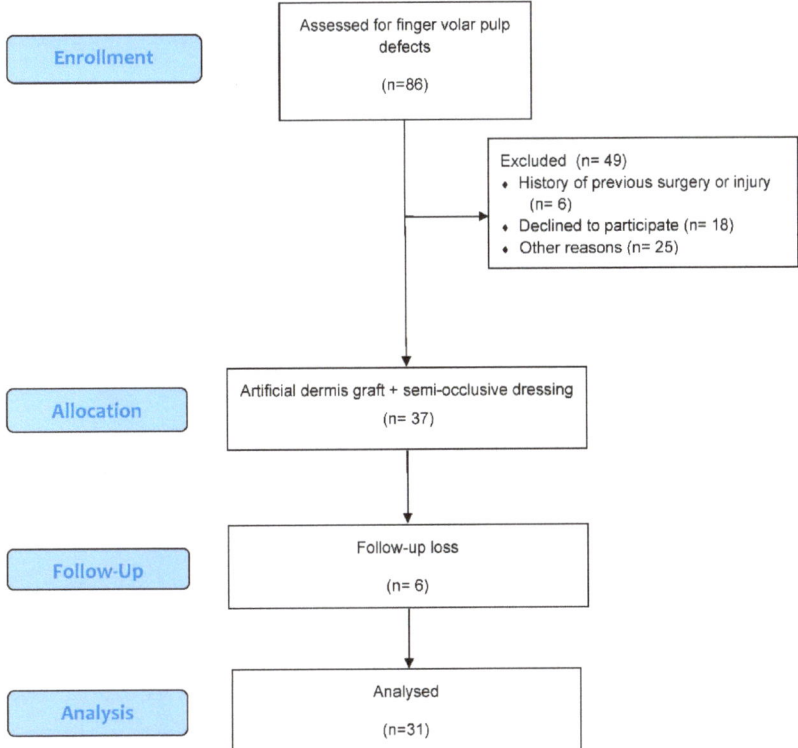

Figure 1. The flow diagram of this study.

2.1. Inclusion and Exclusion Criteria

The inclusion criteria included patients with volar pulp tissue defects who provided informed consent and were unsuitable for immediate replantation. The exclusion criteria were immediate surgical intervention needs, history of surgery or injury to the affected finger, or underlying conditions impairing wound healing.

2.2. Treatment Protocol

All patients underwent wound debridement, irrigation, and hemostasis under digital nerve block in the operating room. The artificial dermis (Pelnac®; Gunze Limited, Kyoto, Japan), a bilayer membrane composed of an outer silicone layer and an inner collagen sponge layer with a thickness of 3 mm, was soaked in saline, trimmed to cover the defect, and secured with 4-0 nylon sutures (Figure 2). A semi-occlusive dressing (IV3000®; Smith & Nephew, Watford, UK), a transparent, waterproof, and breathable polyurethane film dressing, was then applied over the artificial dermis. For patients with excessive oozing, the dressing was changed the following day at the outpatient clinic. In other cases, the first dressing change was performed five days post-operation.

During dressing changes, the finger was soaked in saline for 15 min to minimize damage to the Pelnac® during IV3000® removal. The wound and surrounding area were gently irrigated with saline to prevent infection, and a new IV3000® dressing was applied. The Pelnac® consists of two layers: an inner atelocollagen sponge and an outer silicone layer. After approximately two weeks, the silicone layer was removed, exposing the raw surface. From this point onwards, only the IV3000® dressing was used to cover the wound, creating a moist environment conducive to epithelialization. This process was repeated at five-day intervals until complete epithelialization was achieved, which was defined as the complete coverage of the wound with epithelial tissue without any remaining raw surface. The duration from the initial application of the artificial dermis to complete wound healing was recorded.

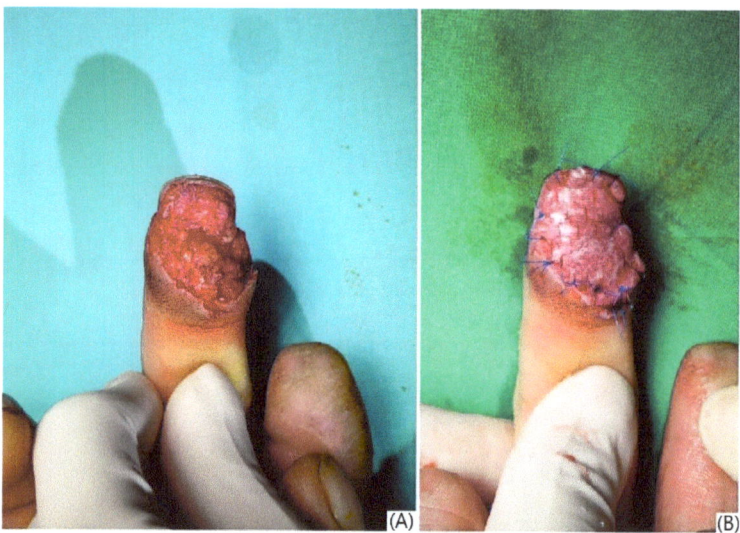

Figure 2. Application of artificial dermis and semi-occlusive dressing for fingertip injury. (**A**) Preoperative view of a middle finger pulp injury; (**B**) intraoperative view showing the application of artificial dermis (Pelnac®) to the defect, followed by a semi-occlusive dressing (IV3000®).

2.3. Outcome Measures

After complete wound healing, patients were asked to complete a subjective questionnaire assessing the following outcomes:

I. Cosmetic satisfaction: rated on a scale from 1 to 5, with higher scores indicating greater satisfaction with the appearance of the treated finger.
II. Sensory impairment: rated on a scale from 0 to 5, with lower scores indicating less sensory loss.
III. Sensory hypersensitivity: rated on a scale from 0 to 5, with lower scores indicating less discomfort or abnormal sensations.
IV. Pain: assessed using a visual analog scale (VAS) ranging from 0 to 5, with lower scores indicating less or no pain.
V. Overall satisfaction: rated on a scale from 1 to 5, with higher scores indicating greater satisfaction with all aspects of the treatment and recovery process.

To objectively evaluate the pulp tissue reconstruction, the degree of fingerprint regeneration was assessed on a scale from 0 to 3, with higher scores indicating better regeneration. This scoring system was developed specifically for this study to quantify the extent of fingerprint recovery: 0 indicating no regeneration, 1 indicating partial regeneration, 2 indicating significant regeneration with some irregularities, and 3 indicating nearly complete regeneration with clear fingerprint patterns.

The outcome assessments were performed by two independent, trained assessors who were blinded to the patients' treatment allocation. The assessors underwent a calibration exercise to ensure consistency and reliability in their evaluations.

Complications, including hook nail deformity and onychomycosis, were recorded throughout the study period. The outcome assessments and follow-up visits were conducted at 1, 3, and 6 months post-treatment.

2.4. Statistical Analysis

The Shapiro–Wilk test was employed to verify the normality of the data distribution. Treatment duration, which followed a normal distribution, was described using means and standard deviations and analyzed using independent sample t-tests to compare:

I. Patients with and without bone exposure.
II. Patients with and without tendon exposure.
III. Patients with both bone and tendon exposure versus those with neither.

Non-normally distributed variables, including fingerprint regeneration scores, cosmetic satisfaction, sensory impairment, sensory hypersensitivity, pain, and overall satisfaction, were described using medians and interquartile ranges. These variables were compared using the Mann–Whitney U test, a non-parametric test, across different patient groups.

Statistical significance was established at a p-value of less than 0.05. All statistical analyses were performed using IBM SPSS Statistics 29.0.2.0 (IBM Corp., Armonk, NY, USA).

3. Results

3.1. Participant Demographics and Injury Characteristics

A total of 31 patients with fingertip injuries were included in this study, conducted between January 2017 and December 2021. The study cohort consisted of 25 males (80.6%) and 6 females (19.4%), with a mean age of 43.29 years (range, 18–72 years). The distribution of the affected fingers is presented in Table 1.

Table 1. Participant demographics and injury characteristics.

Characteristic	Total (N = 31)	Bone Exposure	No Bone Exposure	Tendon Exposure	No Tendon Exposure
Gender					
Male	25 (80.6%)	17	8	8	17
Female	6 (19.4%)	5	1	2	4
Age (years)					
Mean ± SD	43.29 ± 15.00	43.11 ± 17.22	43.36 ± 14.44	40.50 ± 14.73	44.61 ± 15.30
Affected Fingers					
Thumb	3 (9.7%)	2	1	3	0
Index	13 (41.9%)	8	5	8	4
Middle	6 (19.4%)	4	2	4	2
Ring	8 (25.8%)	6	2	4	4
Little	5 (16.1%)	3	2	3	2

Key finding: the study population was predominantly male, and the index finger was the most commonly injured one.

3.2. Treatment Protocol and Healing Duration

Among the 31 patients, 9 (29.03%) had soft tissue injuries without bone exposure, while 22 (70.97%) had injuries with bone exposure (Figure 3). The mean treatment duration for all patients was 45.29 days (SD = 17.53).

Key finding: the mean treatment duration was 45.29 days (SD = 17.53), with no significant differences based on bone or tendon exposure, although cases with tendon exposure required a slightly longer treatment duration compared to those with bone exposure.

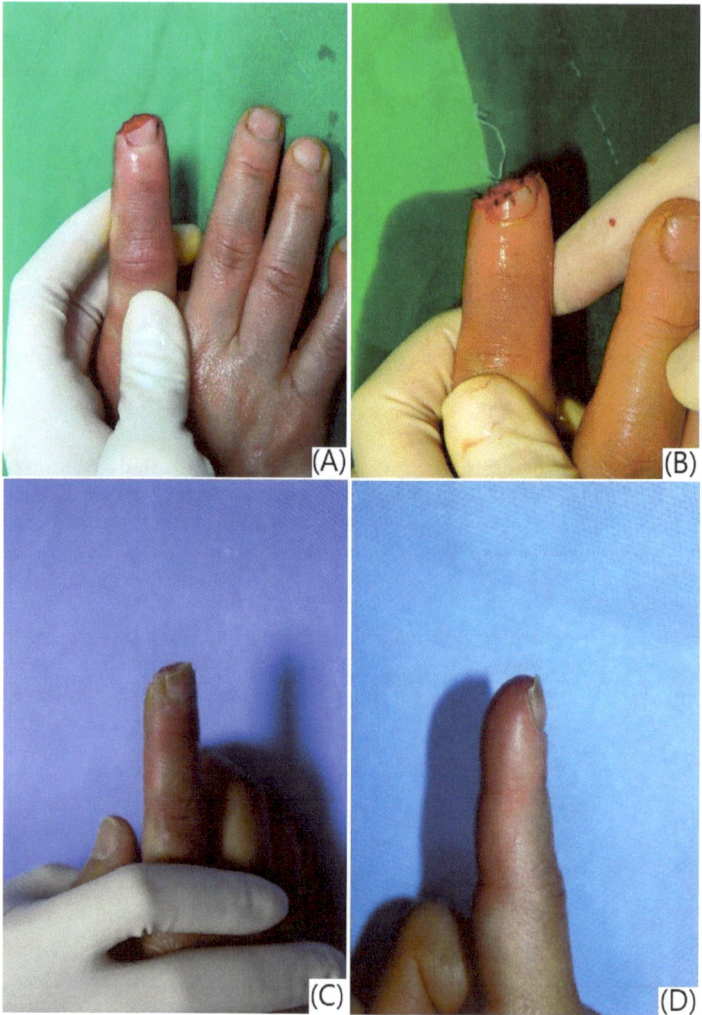

Figure 3. Treatment progression and outcomes following artificial dermis application and semi-occlusive dressing for a fingertip injury. (**A**) Pre-operative view of the right index fingertip injury with distal phalanx and soft tissue defect; (**B**) immediate post-operative view after debridement and application of artificial dermis; (**C**) five weeks post-treatment, showing the regeneration of pulp tissue and early restoration of the fingerprint pattern under the semi-occlusive dressing; (**D**) seven weeks post-treatment, demonstrating complete wound healing with well-formed fingerprint ridges, restored sensation, minimal pain, and satisfactory cosmetic appearance.

3.3. Complications and Clinical Outcomes

Complications were reported in nine patients (29.03%), including hook nail deformity (n = 6, 19.35%), scar contracture (n = 1, 3.22%), onychomycosis (n = 1, 3.22%), and nail splitting (n = 1, 3.22%). Only one complication (3.22%) of nail splitting was directly related to the treatment (Table 2, Figures 4 and 5).

Table 2. Complications and their management.

Complication	No. of Patients (%)	Management
Hook nail deformity	6 (19.35%)	Observation and patient education
Scar contracture	1 (3.22%)	Steroid injection and silicone gel ointment
Onychomycosis	1 (3.22%)	Antifungal medication
Nail splitting	1 (3.22%)	Observation and patient education

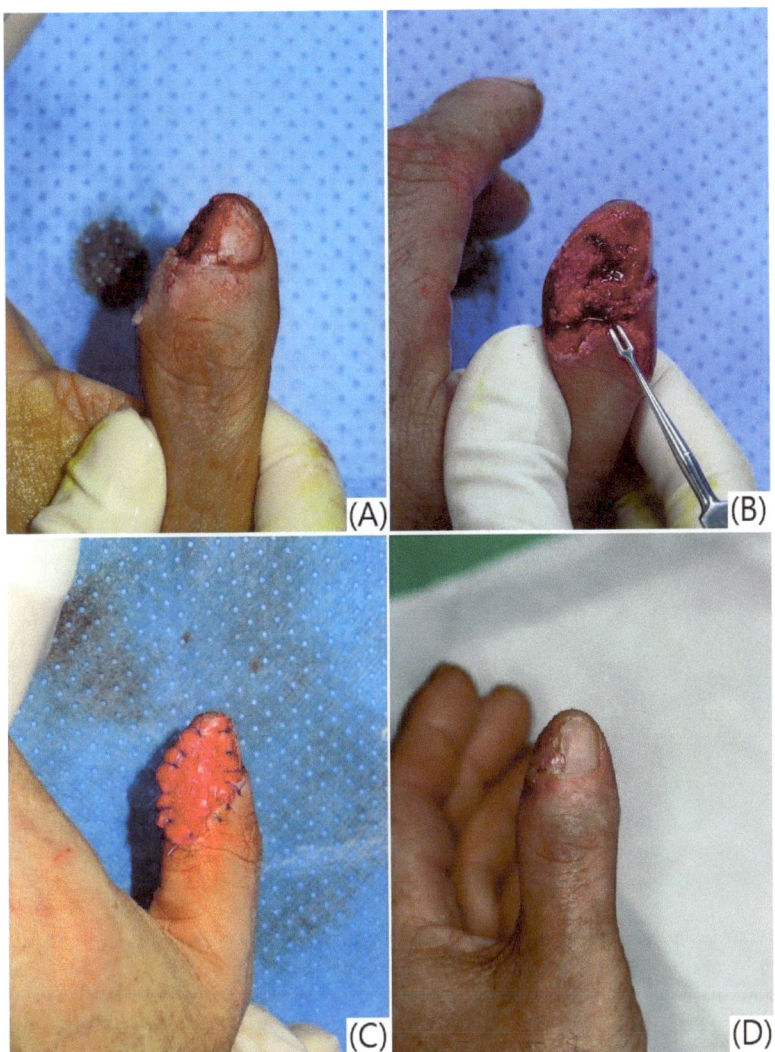

Figure 4. Reconstruction of a thumb tip defect using artificial dermis application and semi-occlusive dressing, resulting in nail splitting. (**A,B**) Pre-operative pictures showing a soft tissue defect of the right thumb side wall with tendon and bone exposure; (**C**) appearance after artificial dermis grafting; (**D**) follow-up photograph 7 weeks after the treatment, demonstrating good healing of the defect site but with observable nail splitting.

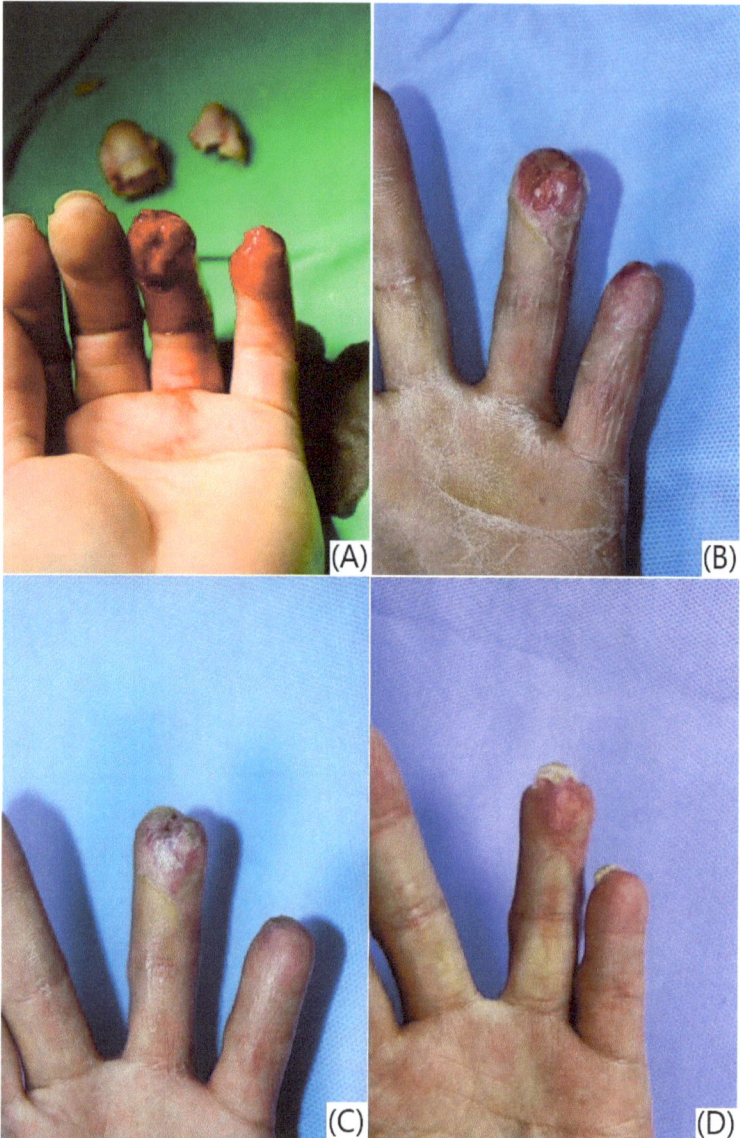

Figure 5. Clinical progression of fingertip regeneration following treatment with artificial dermis and semi-occlusive dressing, demonstrating variability in outcomes. (**A**) Pre-operative view of severe injuries to the left ring and little fingers with complete soft tissue loss and exposed distal phalanges; (**B**) four weeks post-treatment, showing significant granulation tissue formation and coverage of the exposed bone; (**C**) seven weeks post-treatment, demonstrating slower progression of wound healing, with no exposed bone and partial restoration of the fingerprint ridges. However, trophic changes in the nail bed are evident due to the shortened distal phalanges; (**D**) ten weeks post-treatment, revealing complete wound healing with residual scarring on the ring finger and near-complete regeneration of the fingerprint on the little finger. Hook nail deformities are present in both fingers as a consequence of the shortened distal phalanges, which could not be lengthened by the treatment protocol.

Key finding: the treatment demonstrated a low complication rate, with only one case (3.22%) of nail splitting directly attributable to the procedures used in this study.

3.4. Fingerprint Regeneration

The mean fingerprint regeneration score was 2.58 (SD = 0.67) on a scale from 0 to 3, suggesting significant restoration of the fingerprint pattern in most patients.

Key finding: fingerprint regeneration was considerable (mean score = 2.58, SD = 0.67) across all patients, with no statistically significant differences based on bone or tendon exposure (see Table 3 for detailed statistics).

Table 3. Subgroup analysis of outcome measures based on injury characteristics.

Outcome Measure	Bone Exposure	Tendon Exposure	Combined Exposure
Treatment duration (days)	44.11 ± 10.48 (without) vs. 45.77 ± 19.91 (with) (p = 0.131)	41.71 ± 15.67 (without) vs. 52.80 ± 19.65 (with) (p = 0.512)	43.63 ± 11.09 (neither) vs. 53.33 ± 20.76 (both) (p = 0.143)
Fingerprint regeneration score †	2.44 ± 0.88 (without) vs. 2.63 ± 0.58 (with) (p = 0.781)	2.57 ± 0.67 (without) vs. 2.60 ± 0.69 (with) (p = 0.917)	2.37 ± 0.91 (neither) vs. 2.55 ± 0.72 (both) (p = 0.815)
Hypoesthesia score §	0.22 ± 0.66 (without) vs. 0.04 ± 0.21 (with) (p = 0.426)	0.09 ± 0.43 (without) vs. 0.10 ± 0.31 (with) (p = 0.968)	0.25 ± 0.70 (neither) vs. 0.11 ± 0.33 (both) (p = 0.963)
Hyperesthesia score §	0.11 ± 0.33 (without) vs. 0.31 ± 0.64 (with) (p = 0.382)	0.28 ± 0.64 (without) vs. 0.20 ± 0.42 (with) (p = 0.702)	0.12 ± 0.35 (neither) vs. 0.22 ± 0.44 (both) (p = 0.743)
Pain score (VAS) §	0.44 ± 0.52 (without) vs. 0.45 ± 0.73 (with) (p = 0.781)	0.38 ± 0.58 (without) vs. 0.60 ± 0.84 (with) (p = 0.633)	0.37 ± 0.51 (neither) vs. 0.55 ± 0.88 (both) (p = 0.743)
Cosmetic satisfaction score ¶	4.22 ± 0.97 (without) vs. 4.04 ± 0.95 (with) (p = 0.654)	4.14 ± 0.91 (without) vs. 4.00 ± 1.05 (with) (p = 0.787)	4.12 ± 0.99 (neither) vs. 3.88 ± 1.05 (both) (p = 0.673)
Overall satisfaction score ¶	4.66 ± 0.70 (without) vs. 4.31 ± 0.64 (with) (p = 0.174)	4.47 ± 0.67 (without) vs. 4.30 ± 0.67 (with) (p = 0.492)	4.62 ± 0.74 (neither) vs. 4.22 ± 0.66 (both) (p = 0.236)

Data presented as without exposure vs. with exposure, p > 0.05 for all comparisons (independent samples t-test). † Assessed on a scale from 0 to 3, with higher scores indicating better regeneration. Data presented as without exposure vs. with exposure, p > 0.05 for all comparisons (Mann–Whitney U test). § Rated on a scale from 0 to 5, with lower scores indicating less sensory loss, discomfort or pain. ¶ Rated on a scale from 1 to 5, with higher scores indicating greater satisfaction.

3.5. Sensory Assessment

3.5.1. Hypoesthesia

The mean hypoesthesia score for all 31 patients was 0.09 (SD = 0.39), indicating minimal sensory deficits.

Key finding: hypoesthesia was minimal (mean = 0.09, SD = 0.39), with no significant differences across various injury types.

3.5.2. Hyperesthesia

The mean hyperesthesia score for all 31 patients was 0.25 (SD = 0.57), indicating minimal sensory disturbances.

Key finding: hyperesthesia was minimal (mean = 0.25, SD = 0.57), with no significant differences across various injury types.

3.6. Pain Assessment

The mean pain score for all 31 patients was 0.45 (SD = 0.67), indicating minimal post-treatment pain.

Key finding: post-treatment pain was minimal (mean = 0.45, SD = 0.67), with no significant differences across various injury types.

3.7. Cosmetic Assessment

The mean cosmetic satisfaction score for all 31 patients was 4.09 (SD = 0.94), indicating high satisfaction with the cosmetic outcomes.

Key finding: cosmetic satisfaction was high (mean = 4.09, SD = 0.94), with no significant differences across various injury types.

3.8. Overall Satisfaction

The mean overall satisfaction score for all 31 patients was 4.41 (SD = 0.67), indicating high satisfaction with the treatment outcomes.

Key finding: overall treatment satisfaction was high (mean = 4.41, SD = 0.67), with no significant differences across various injury types (Table 3).

4. Discussion

This prospective study demonstrates the efficacy of a conservative treatment protocol combining artificial dermis (Pelnac®) and semi-occlusive dressings (IV3000®) in managing fingertip injuries with volar pulp tissue defects. The findings underscore the potential of this synergistic approach for achieving favorable clinical outcomes while minimizing surgical morbidity and hospitalization, aligning with the growing emphasis on patient-centered care in reconstructive surgery [27,28].

The study cohort exhibited substantial fingerprint regeneration, with slightly better scores in patients with bone-exposed injuries. This improvement could be attributed to the regenerative capabilities of the periosteum and bone marrow cells, as well as the inflammatory response triggering the recruitment of mesenchymal stem cells and growth factors [29,30]. These findings suggest that the conservative treatment protocol, which harnesses the body's inherent regenerative mechanisms, may be particularly beneficial for patients with bone-exposed fingertip injuries.

The treatment duration in the current study (45.29 days, SD = 17.53) was slightly longer than those reported by Namgoong et al. [18] and Wang et al. [12], who also used artificial dermis for fingertip defects with bone exposure. This prolonged duration may be attributed to the unique combination of artificial dermis and semi-occlusive dressing, which likely influences the complex regenerative processes within the wound bed. Despite the longer treatment duration, the current study achieved high patient satisfaction, good sensory recovery, and favorable cosmetic outcomes, consistent with the key outcomes reported in other studies (Table 4). However, the heterogeneity in study designs, sample sizes, and specific interventions among these studies makes direct comparisons challenging.

The consistently low pain levels across all subgroups suggest effective pain management by the treatment protocol, possibly due to the anti-inflammatory properties of the artificial dermis and the protective barrier provided by the semi-occlusive dressing [31]. However, the conclusion of a "low pain level" should be interpreted cautiously, as the sensory evaluation was conducted immediately after epithelialization and may not fully capture long-term pain levels and nerve recovery [32].

This study has several limitations that warrant careful consideration. First, the absence of a surgical control group may affect the generalizability of the findings. This decision was guided by multiple factors: the inherent drawbacks of surgical interventions [6–8,10,13,33], encouraging outcomes from conservative approaches in prior studies [12,14,16,17,21–24,34–36], and significant recruitment challenges due to patients' strong preference for less invasive treatments [37]. Moreover, based on the author's experience, the toe pulp free flap was identified as the most comparable surgical technique to the proposed conservative treatment. However, its inclusion in this study was impractical given the highly specialized nature of the procedure and the significantly lower number of eligible patients, making it unfeasible to create a control group for this technique.

Table 4. Comparison of treatment duration with previous studies utilizing artificial dermis for fingertip reconstruction.

Study	Sample Size	Injury Type	Method	Treatment Duration (days)	Key Outcomes
Current Study	31	Volar pulp defects with bone and/or tendon exposure	Pelnac®	45.29 ± 17.53	High patient satisfaction, good sensory recovery, and cosmetic outcomes
Wang et al., 2022 [12]	24	Fingertip defects with bone exposure	Pelnac®	28~42	Improves appearance and function, and decreases the need for stump trimming in amputated fingers.
Namgoong et al., 2020 [18]	23	Fingertip defects with bone exposure	Tissue-engineered artificial dermis	34.0 ± 4.9	Superior functional and aesthetic outcome compared to artificial dermis graft
Hoigné et al., 2014 [23]	19	Fingertip amputations (Ishikawa zones II–III)	OpSite® Flexifix® (Richardson Healthcare Ltd., Borehamwood, UK) dressing	21~56	Good sensory recovery and cosmetic outcomes
Boudard et al., 2019 [38]	19	Fingertip amputations (M and D * zones I–III)	Semi-occlusive dressing (Tegaderm®, 3M Company, St. Paul, MN, USA)	30.1 ± 7	Good functional and cosmetic outcomes
Mennen and Wiese, 1993 [36]	200	Various fingertip injuries	Semi-occlusive dressing (OpSite®)	20–30	Good functional and cosmetic outcomes, low complication rate

* M & D: Merle and Dautel.

Another important limitation is the lack of objective sensory recovery assessments, such as the two-point discrimination test, which could have provided a more comprehensive evaluation of sensory outcomes [39]. Additionally, the relatively short follow-up period restricts the ability to fully assess the long-term durability and efficacy of the treatment. Addressing these limitations in future research will be crucial for validating and extending the findings of this study.

To address these limitations and further advance the understanding of conservative approaches for managing fingertip injuries, future research should focus on the following areas:

1. Conducting well-designed, randomized controlled trials comparing conservative treatments with surgical interventions, using standardized outcome measures and longer follow-up periods to assess long-term efficacy, durability, pain levels, and nerve recovery.
2. Performing comparative studies on different dermal substitutes and dressing materials to identify the most effective combinations that minimize treatment time while maximizing regenerative outcomes.
3. Incorporating objective sensory assessments, such as the two-point discrimination test, alongside subjective evaluations to provide a more comprehensive understanding of sensory recovery

5. Conclusions

This study demonstrates the potential of a novel conservative treatment protocol combining artificial dermis and semi-occlusive dressings in managing fingertip injuries with volar pulp tissue defects. Despite its limitations, such as the absence of a surgical control group and the relatively short follow-up period, the approach achieves favorable clinical outcomes while minimizing surgical morbidity and aligning with patient-centered care principles. The results suggest that this synergistic combination may offer a promising alternative to traditional surgical interventions for managing fingertip injuries, particularly in patients with bone-exposed defects. However, further research with longer follow-up periods, objective sensory assessments, and comparative studies is needed to establish the long-term efficacy, durability, and superiority of this approach over existing surgical techniques.

Funding: This research received no external funding.

Institutional Review Board Statement: This single-center, prospective study was approved by the Institutional Review Board of the Catholic Kwandong University International St. Mary's Hospital (IRB No. 19 year IRB069, Registration No. IS19EISE0072). All procedures followed were in accordance with the ethical standards of the responsible committee on human experimentation (institutional and national) and with the Helsinki Declaration of 1975, as revised in 2008. Informed consent was obtained from all patients for being included in this study.

Informed Consent Statement: Informed consent was obtained from all subjects involved in this study.

Data Availability Statement: The data presented in this study are not publicly available due to privacy and ethical restrictions, as the research involves sensitive patient information.

Conflicts of Interest: The author declares no conflicts of interest.

References

1. Martin-Playa, P.; Foo, A. Approach to Fingertip Injuries. *Clin. Plast. Surg.* **2019**, *46*, 275–283. [CrossRef]
2. Farahani, R.M.; Simonian, M.; Hunter, N. Blueprint of an ancestral neurosensory organ revealed in glial networks in human dental pulp. *J. Comp. Neurol.* **2011**, *519*, 3306–3326. [CrossRef]
3. Karthi Sundar, V.; Gandhi, B.S.; Sundaram, P.S. Surgical management of fingertip injuries. *Int. J. Res. Orthop.* **2017**, *3*, 19.
4. Lin, J.; Wang, J.; Hu, D.; Xu, Y.; Zhang, T. *Reconstruction of Finger Pulp Defects*, in Atlas of Finger Reconstruction: Techniques and Cases; Springer Nature Singapore: Singapore, 2023; pp. 225–244.
5. Zeng, Q. Reverse Homodigital Artery Island Flap with Palmar Cutaneous Branches of the Proper Digital Nerve for Repairing of Finger Pulp Defect and Sensory Reconstruction: Is It Deserving? *Ann. Plast. Surg.* **2023**, *91*, 789. [CrossRef]
6. Zhang, X.; Wang, Z.; Ma, X.; Jin, Y.; Wang, J.; Yu, H.; Li, T.; Xiu, X. Repair of finger pulp defects using a free second toe pulp flap anastomosed with the palmar vein. *J. Orthop. Surg. Res.* **2022**, *17*, 352. [CrossRef]
7. Wang, S.; Yuan, C.; Ding, W.; Shen, H.; Gu, J. Repair of finger pulp defect and sensory reconstruction using reverse homodigital artery island flap with palmar cutaneous branches of the proper digital nerve. *Ann. Plast. Surg.* **2023**, *90*, 559–563. [CrossRef] [PubMed]
8. Troisi, L.M.; Zanchetta, F.; Berner, J.E.M.; Mosillo, G.; Pajardi, G.E. Reconstruction of digital defects with the free proximal ulnar artery perforator flap. *Plast. Reconstr. Surg.—Glob. Open* **2022**, *10*, e4054. [CrossRef] [PubMed]
9. Nakanishi, A.; Omokawa, S.; Kawamura, K.; Iida, A.; Kaji, D.; Tanaka, Y. Tamai zone 1 fingertip amputation: Reconstruction using a digital artery flap compared with microsurgical replantation. *J. Hand Surg.* **2019**, *44*, 655–661. [CrossRef]
10. Panattoni, J.B.; De Ona, I.R.; Ahmed, M.M. Reconstruction of fingertip injuries: Surgical tips and avoiding complications. *J. Hand Surg.* **2015**, *40*, 1016–1024. [CrossRef]
11. Rautio, S.B.; Paukkunen, A.; Jokihaara, J. A Prospective Follow-up Study of Fingertip Amputation Treatment with Semi-occlusive Dressing. *Plast. Reconstr. Surg.—Glob. Open* **2023**, *11*, e5407. [CrossRef]
12. Wang, J.; Huang, Z.; Jumbo, J.C.C.; Sha, K. Long-term follow-up of one-stage artificial dermis reconstruction surgery for fingertip defects with exposed phalanx. *Hand Surg. Rehabil.* **2022**, *41*, 353–361. [CrossRef]
13. Nakanishi, A.; Kawamura, K.; Omokawa, S.; Hasegawa, H.; Tanaka, Y. Clinical outcomes of reposition flap transfer for fingertip amputation. *Eur. J. Orthop. Surg. Traumatol.* **2024**, *34*, 1627–1634. [CrossRef] [PubMed]
14. Balagué, N.; L'Huillier, A.G. Regenerative healing ability of the digit tip. *J. Am. Acad. Dermatol.* **2023**, *88*, e185–e186. [CrossRef] [PubMed]
15. Wosgrau, A.C.C.; Jeremias, T.D.S.; Leonardi, D.F.; Pereima, M.J.; Di Giunta, G.; Trentin, A.G. Comparative experimental study of wound healing in mice: Pelnac versus Integra. *PLoS ONE* **2015**, *10*, e0120322. [CrossRef] [PubMed]
16. Hamdan, A.M.; Al-Chalabi, M.M.M.; Sulaiman, W.A.W. Integra: An Alternative Option for Reconstruction of Extensive Finger Defects with Exposed Bones. *Cureus* **2021**, *13*, e16223. [CrossRef] [PubMed]
17. Lou, X.; Xue, H.; Li, G.; Wang, K.; Zhou, P.; Li, B.; Chen, J. One-stage Pelnac Reconstruction in Full-thickness Skin Defects with Bone or Tendon Exposure. *Plast. Reconstr. Surg.—Glob. Open* **2018**, *6*, e1709. [CrossRef] [PubMed]
18. Namgoong, S.M.; Jung, J.E.; Han, S.-K.M.; Jeong, S.-H.M.; Dhong, E.-S.M. Potential of Tissue-Engineered and Artificial Dermis Grafts for Fingertip Reconstruction. *Plast. Reconstr. Surg.* **2020**, *146*, 1082–1095. [CrossRef] [PubMed]
19. Watt, F.M.; Fujiwara, H. Cell-extracellular matrix interactions in normal and diseased skin. *Cold Spring Harb. Perspect. Biol.* **2011**, *3*, a005124. [CrossRef] [PubMed]

20. Wu, Y.; Huang, C.; Zhang, X.; Shen, G. The clinical application effects of artificial dermis scaffold and autologous split-thickness skin composite grafts combined with vacuum-assisted closure in refractory wounds. *Int. Wound J.* **2023**, *20*, 2113–2120. [CrossRef]
21. Mensah, R.A.; Jo, S.B.; Kim, H.; Park, S.M.; Patel, K.D.; Cho, K.J.; Cook, M.T.; Kirton, S.B.; Hutter, V.; Sidney, L.E.; et al. The eggshell membrane: A potential biomaterial for corneal wound healing. *J. Biomater. Appl.* **2021**, *36*, 912–929. [CrossRef]
22. Pastor, T.; Hermann, P.; Haug, L.; Gueorguiev, B.; Pastor, T.; Vögelin, E. Semi-occlusive dressing therapy versus surgical treatment in fingertip amputation injuries: A clinical study. *Eur. J. Trauma Emerg. Surg.* **2023**, *49*, 1441–1447. [CrossRef] [PubMed]
23. Hoigné, D.; Hug, U.; Schürch, M.; Meoli, M.; von Wartburg, U. Semi-occlusive dressing for the treatment of fingertip amputations with exposed bone: Quantity and quality of soft-tissue regeneration. *J. Hand Surg. Eur. Vol.* **2013**, *39*, 505–509. [CrossRef] [PubMed]
24. Schultz, J.; Wruck, J.E.; Trips, E.; Pfeiffer, R.; Grählert, X.; Münchow, S.; Schröttner, P.; Dragu, A.; Fitze, G. Semi-occlusive management of fingertip injuries with finger caps: A randomized controlled trial in children and adults. *Medicine* **2022**, *101*, e29324. [CrossRef]
25. Lin, Y.-N.; Wang, Y.-C.; Lee, S.-S.; Hsieh, M.-C.W.; Lin, S.-D.; Huang, S.-H.; Lin, T.-M.; Kuo, Y.-R. The bridging effect of artificial dermis on reconstruction of skin avulsion injury. *Int. J. Low. Extrem. Wounds*, 2023; *Online ahead of print*. [CrossRef]
26. Han, S.-K. Biologic Dermis Graft. In *Innovations and Advances in Wound Healing*; Springer: Berlin/Heidelberg, Germany, 2023; pp. 77–96.
27. Hutchison, A.M.; Bodger, O.; Whelan, R.; Russell, I.D.; Man, W.; Williams, P.; Bebbington, A. Functional outcome and patient satisfaction with a 'self-care' protocol for minimally displaced distal radius fractures: A service evaluation. *Bone Jt. Open* **2022**, *3*, 726–732. [CrossRef]
28. De Ridder, W.A.; Wouters, R.M.; Hoogendam, L.; Vermeulen, G.M.; Slijper, H.P.; Selles, R.W. Which factors are associated with satisfaction with treatment results in patients with hand and wrist conditions? A large cohort analysis. *Clin. Orthop. Relat. Res.* **2022**, *480*, 1287–1301. [CrossRef]
29. Zhang, X.; Li, J.; Ye, P.; Gao, G.; Hubbell, K.; Cui, X. Coculture of mesenchymal stem cells and endothelial cells enhances host tissue integration and epidermis maturation through AKT activation in gelatin methacryloyl hydrogel-based skin model. *Acta Biomater.* **2017**, *59*, 317–326. [CrossRef]
30. Leitão, L.; Neto, E.; Conceição, F.; Monteiro, A.; Couto, M.; Alves, C.J.; Sousa, D.M.; Lamghari, M. Osteoblasts are inherently programmed to repel sensory innervation. *Bone Res.* **2020**, *8*, 20. [CrossRef]
31. Junker, J.P.; Kamel, R.A.; Caterson, E.; Eriksson, E. Clinical impact upon wound healing and inflammation in moist, wet, and dry environments. *Adv. Wound Care* **2013**, *2*, 348–356. [CrossRef] [PubMed]
32. Mukhtar, R.; Fazal, M.U.; Saleem, M.; Saleem, S. Role of low-level laser therapy in post-herpetic neuralgia: A pilot study. *Lasers Med. Sci.* **2020**, *35*, 1759–1764. [CrossRef]
33. Ryang, S.-R.; Jang, M.-G.; Kim, K.-C.; Gun, S. Clinical Study on Reconstruction of Soft Tissue Defects of the Digits by Volar Flaps. *J. Orthop. Sports Med.* **2020**, *2*, 10–17. [CrossRef]
34. Cheang, C.J.Y.; Khan, M.A.A.; Jordan, D.J.; Nassar, K.; Bhatti, D.S.; Rafiq, S.; Hogg, F.J.; Waterston, S.W. IV3000 semi-occlusive dressing use in simple and complex fingertip injuries: Efficacy and affordability. *J. Wound Care* **2022**, *31*, 340–347. [CrossRef] [PubMed]
35. Quadlbauer, S.; Pezzei, C.; Beer, T.; Hausner, T.; Leixnering, M. Therapy of Fingertip Injuries: The Semiocclusive Dressing as an Alternative Option to Local Skin Flaps. *HAND* **2016**, *11* (Suppl. S1), 60S. [CrossRef]
36. Mennen, U.; Wiese, A. Fingertip Injuries Management with Semiocclusive Dressing. *J. Hand Surg.* **1993**, *18*, 416–422. [CrossRef] [PubMed]
37. van Werkhoven, E.; Tajik, P.; Bossuyt, P.M. Always randomize as late as possible. *Gastric Cancer* **2019**, *22*, 1308–1309. [CrossRef] [PubMed]
38. Boudard, J.; Loisel, F.; El Rifaï, S.; Feuvrier, D.; Obert, L.; Pluvy, I. Fingertip amputations treated with occlusive dressingsAmputation digitale distale traitée par pansement occlusif. *Hand Surg. Rehabil.* **2019**, *38*, 257–261. [CrossRef]
39. Huber, J.; Scharberth, A.; Maier, C.; Wallner, C.M.; Wagner, J.M.; Dadras, M.; Longaker, M.T.M.; Lehnhardt, M.; Behr, B. Standardized Quantitative Sensory Testing to Assess Insufficient Recovery of Touch Discrimination in Free Flap Surgery. *Plast. Reconstr. Surg.* **2022**, *151*, 429–438. [CrossRef]

Disclaimer/Publisher's Note: The statements, opinions and data contained in all publications are solely those of the individual author(s) and contributor(s) and not of MDPI and/or the editor(s). MDPI and/or the editor(s) disclaim responsibility for any injury to people or property resulting from any ideas, methods, instructions or products referred to in the content.

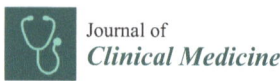

Article

Surgical Navigation and CAD-CAM-Designed PEEK Prosthesis for the Surgical Treatment of Facial Intraosseous Vascular Anomalies

Alicia Dean [1,*], Orlando Estévez [1], Concepción Centella [1], Alba Sanjuan-Sanjuan [2], Marina E. Sánchez-Frías [3] and Francisco J. Alamillos [1]

[1] Maxillofacial Surgery Department, Reina Sofía University Hospital, Maimonides Institute for Biomedical Research of Córdoba (IMIBIC), 14004 Cordoba, Spain; orlando_estevez@hotmail.com (O.E.); centellaguti@hotmail.com (C.C.); drfalami@gmail.com (F.J.A.)
[2] Maxillofacial Surgery Department, Charleston Area Medical Center, Charleston, WV 25301, USA; albasanjuan@hotmail.com
[3] Pathology Department, Reina Sofía University Hospital, Maimonides Institute for Biomedical Research of Córdoba (IMIBIC), 14004 Cordoba, Spain; marinasanchezfrias@gmail.com
* Correspondence: adeanferrer@yahoo.es

Abstract: Background: Intraosseous vascular anomalies in the facial skeleton present significant diagnostic and therapeutic challenges due to complex anatomy. These anomalies represent about 0.5–1% of bony neoplastic and tumor-like lesions, usually presenting as a firm, painless mass. Most described intraosseous vascular malformations are venous malformations (VMs) and, more rarely, arteriovenous malformations. **Objectives**: The objectives of this work are to show our experience, protocol and the applications of computer planning, virtual surgery, CAD-CAM design, surgical navigation, and computer-assisted navigated piezoelectric surgery in the treatment of facial intraosseous vascular anomalies and to evaluate the advantages and disadvantages. **Methods**: Three females and one male with periorbital intraosseous vascular anomalies were treated using en-block resection and immediate reconstruction with a custom-made PEEK prosthesis. One lesion was in the supraorbital rim and orbital roof, one in the frontal bone and orbital roof, and two in the zygomatic region. We accomplished the resection and reconstruction of the lesion using virtual planning, CAD-CAM design, surgical navigation and piezoelectric device navigation. **Results**: There were no complications related to the surgery assisted with navigation. With an accuracy of less than 1 mm, the procedure may be carried out in accordance with the surgical plan. The surgeon's degree of uncertainty during deep osteotomies and in locations with low visibility was decreased by the use of the navigated piezoelectric device. **Conclusions**: Resection and reconstruction of facial intraosseous vascular anomalies benefit from this new surgical strategy using CAD-CAM technologies, computer-assisted navigated piezoelectric surgery, and surgical navigation.

Keywords: surgical navigation; virtual surgery; CAD-CAM design; computed-assisted surgery; virtual planning; computer-assisted navigated piezoelectric surgery; 3D planning

1. Introduction

Intraosseous vascular anomalies of the facial skeleton present a significant diagnostic and therapeutic challenge due to its complex anatomy [1].

According to Mulliken and Glowacki, there are two types of vascular anomalies: vascular tumors and vascular malformations [2]. The 2018 International Society for the Study of Vascular Anomalies (ISSVA) classification does not accept the diagnosis of intraosseous hemangioma, distinguishing between proliferative lesions (tumors) and non-proliferative lesions (malformations) [3–5].

Most described intraosseous vascular malformations are venous malformations (VMs) and more rarely arteriovenous malformations (AVMs). Many have been erroneously labeled as "hemangiomas" [1,5].

These anomalies represent about 0.5–1% of all bony neoplastic and tumor-like lesions and mostly affect the vertebral column and calvarium [6,7]. Maxillofacial involvement is uncommon, with the maxilla and mandible being the most frequently affected sites [6–8]. Zygomatic bone, nasal, and frontal bone involvement has also been described [9–12].

They typically occur in the fourth to fifth decade, affecting both genders almost equally [5,7], although some studies note a female predominance [6,9]. Trauma is a commonly suggested cause [13–15], although congenital factors are also considered [16–18]. VMs present as a firm, painless lump or mass [1,7,19,20] and can cause swelling or pain in the maxilla and the mandible, or neurological symptoms when in the sphenoid bone [21] or cranial base [22,23]. Rarely, they can cause tooth displacement [7]. Lesions of periorbital bones usually produce asymptomatic contour defects with esthetic compromise [6,8,10,24–26]. When symptomatic, pain (49%) and subsequent by ocular features (14.2%) related to the mass effect (dystopia, exorbitism, ptosis and extraocular muscle movement impairment) are the most common symptoms [9,25,27–33].

VMs show a tendency to grow with time and can worsen due to trauma, infection, puberty or pregnancy [7,11,34]. Traumatic injury may predispose to periods of accelerated growth; however, this association remains controversial [6].

There may be extensive bleeding during biopsy or surgery; so, it is imperative to suspect the vascular nature of the lesion [9].

On plain radiography, VMs are slightly radiopaque and usually well circumscribed [35]. On CT, the lesions may appear with honeycomb, soap bubble, or sunburst patterns [6,15,18,28,34–37]. On MRI, VMs appear hypo- to isointense on T1 images and hyperintense on T2 images. In orthopantomography and plain radiography, AVMs appear as radiolucent lesions, and CT scans show them as expansive lytic defects that are vividly enhanced on contrast administration [35,38]. On MRI, an AVM appears as a tangle of vessels with a typical flow–void phenomenon, seen on both T1- and T2-weighted imaging [1,29,34,38]. CT is the standard radiological study. However, several authors prefer MRI to CT [13,18,39].

Histopathology differentiates VMs, characterized by abnormal thin-walled veins, from AVMs, with arteriovenous shunts [6].

Immunohistochemical staining also aids in distinguishing these lesions: VMs are positive for CD31 and CD34, AVMs for smooth muscle actin, and hemangiomas for GLUT-1 [6].

Treatment depends on symptoms, location, and extent.

Complete surgical resection is its treatment of choice [7,8,19,24,40], reducing recurrence [40], and bleeding risks [9,26]. Preoperative arteriography and embolization may be beneficial for high-flow lesions.

Advanced technologies like virtual planning, surgical navigation, and computer-assisted navigated piezoelectric surgery (CANPS) enhance precision and outcomes and minimize complications and surgical approaches in the surgical treatment of facial intraosseous vascular anomalies [41–47].

Computer-assisted navigated piezoelectric surgery (CANPS) applies computer planning and surgical navigation to a piezoelectric device so that it becomes navigable [48,49].

The main objective of this work is to show our experience, our protocol, and the applications of computer planning, virtual surgery, CAD-CAM design, surgical navigation and computer-assisted navigated piezoelectric surgery in the treatment of facial intraosseous vascular anomalies and to evaluate the advantages and disadvantages of this innovative surgical approach.

2. Materials and Methods

2.1. Patients

The study design is based on a descriptive study (case series) of 4 patients with intraosseous vascular anomalies treated in the Department of Craniomaxillofacial Surgery at a tertiary referral hospital between June 2017 and May 2019. All patients provided informed written consent to accomplish the surgery and posteriorly also to participate in the study.

The inclusion criteria were as follows: (1) presence of a craniomaxillofacial intraosseous vascular anomaly; (2) resection and reconstruction of the tumor using virtual planning, CAD-CAM design and surgical navigation; and (3) minimum follow-up of 1 year. The exclusion criteria were as follows: (1) resection of intraosseous vascular anomaly without virtual planning, CAD-CAM design and surgical navigation; and (2) incomplete records.

2.2. Data Collection

Data collection was carried out based on a protocol established before the study began and reviewed at the end of it. Clinical variables related to the patients were recorded. The variables and data collection form are attached in Table 1.

2.3. Procedure

En-block resection and immediate custom-made PEEK prosthesis reconstruction were planned for all four patients.

2.3.1. Virtual Surgical Plan

DICOM (Digital Imaging and Communication in Medicine) files from CT helical scan with 0.8 mm thin slices data were imported into the planning BrainLab software, iPlan® 3.0.6 and Elements® 4.0 (Munich, Germany). A virtual surgery with a treatment plan was carried out. The vascular malformation shape was outlined, and an appropriate 1mm surgical margin was automatically created using the tool "margin". The object "lesion resection" was created and the virtual bone defect was evaluated after the virtual resection was performed on the computer. Essential anatomical structures to be protected from injury during surgery were also delimited and marked.

2.3.2. CAD-CAM Design of the PEEK Prosthesis

The object "lesion resection" was converted into .STL files that were sent to Materialise® (Materialise, Leuven, Belgium; https://www.materialise.com/en, accessed on 31 July 2024), which built a custom-made PEEK prosthesis. The prosthesis was manufactured by mirroring the healthy side and following surgical resection margins. The surgical plan, resection guide, and prosthesis were converted into .STL files. The files were sent back to us and imported into the iPlan® 3.05 software or Elements® planning software of the BrainLab® navigation system. The .STL files of the plan were superimposed onto patient-specific CT scan data to check the accuracy of the resection and PEEK reconstruction plan.

Table 1. Patient data, clinical symptoms, locations, histopathology, virtual surgery, surgical navigation, reconstruction.

Case	Age/Sex	Side/Size	Pain	Time of Evolution	Ocular Symptoms	History of Trauma	Imaging	Localization	Histopathology	GLUT-1	Treatment	Virtual Planning	Surgical Navigation	Type of Surgical Navigation	Surgical Approach	Surgical Guides	Surgical Device (Bone Resection)	Bleeding	Reconstruction	Follow-Up/Recurrence
1	53/F	L/25 mm	Y	4 mo	Dystopia	N	CT, MRI	Supraorbital rim, orbital roof	Intraosseous venous malformation	-	Resection + reconstruction	Y	Y	1st, 2nd, 3rd	Coronal	Y	Piezoelectric device	N	PEEK prosthesis	7 y/N
2	54/F	R/33 mm	Y	9 y	N	Y	CT, MRI	Frontal bone, orbital roof	Intraosseous venous malformation	-	Resection + reconstruction	Y	Y	1st, 2nd, 3rd	Coronal	Y	Piezoelectric device	N	PEEK prosthesis	6 y/N
3	36/F	L/19 mm	Y	6 mo	N	N	CT, MRI	Zygoma	Arteriovenous malformation	-	Resection + reconstruction	Y	Y	1st, 2nd, 3rd	Transconjunctival + blepharoplasty + maxillary vestibular	Y	Piezoelectric device	N	PEEK prosthesis	5 y/N
4	47/M	L/30 mm	N	2 y	N	N	CT	Zygoma	Intraosseous venous malformation	-	Resection + reconstruction	Y	Y	1st, 2nd, 3rd	Transconjunctival + lateral canthotomy + maxillary vestibular	Y	Piezoelectric device	N	PEEK prosthesis	6 y/N

Abbreviations: F, female; M, male; CT, computed tomography; MRI, magnetic resonance imaging; mo, month; y, year; Y, yes; N, no; 1st, first navigation; 2nd, second navigation; 3rd, third navigation.

2.3.3. Surgical Navigation

Surgical navigation with the BrainLab® system was used to guide the resection. There are three moments of surgical navigation: anatomical navigation (1st navigation), working navigation (2nd navigation), and checking navigation (3rd navigation). Anatomical navigation checks anatomical structures, working navigation helps with surgical plans, and checking navigation or simulation-guided navigation verifies reconstruction [49,50]. CANPS is a type of working navigation [49,50].

A skull post with a dynamic reference frame was fixed to the patient's skull. Patient registration was performed using the surface laser or unequivocal bone points.

Registration and calibration of the cutting tip of the piezoelectric device were carried out. The piezoelectric handpiece was registered by anchoring the three reflecting spheres tracking tool to the handpiece of a Vercellotti-type piezoelectric device and linking it to the navigator with a calibration matrix. The cutting guides were set in position and anchored with screws onto the healthy bone. The osteotomy of the lesion was performed with a piezoelectric device following the custom-made surgical guides over the bone surface and then in depth in the orbital roof, orbital floor and orbital walls with the aid of the CANPS. We accomplished 1. Indirect, and 2. Direct or "live" surgical navigation. We performed live piezoelectric navigation with real-time results on the workstation screen. The precision of the piezoelectric device's cutting tip was monitored before and throughout the surgery. Accuracy was ensured by positioning the calibrated cutting tip on specific anatomical landmarks. Surgery was carried out with a precision of 1 mm. If deviations exceeded this limit, the device was re-registered and recalibrated. After the resection, the navigation again helped us check the planned resection margins.

The PEEK prostheses were placed in position for reconstruction. Patient-specific implants did not require additional adaptation or remodeling because navigation-assisted resection ensured precise excision of the deep margins according to the preoperative plan. In Case 1, a groove was created for the passage of the pericranial flap to isolate the frontal sinus and nasal cavities from the skull base and prosthesis. This groove, approximately 3 mm thick, prevents compression over the pericranial flap when placing the PEEK prosthesis. The customized PEEK prostheses were fixed in all cases with titanium mini-plates. Osteosynthesis was performed using conventional osteosynthesis systems (Matrix Midface®) with low-profile mini-plates to prevent them from being palpable under the skin. Two holes and screws at least on each side of the osteosynthesis points were used. Navigation was performed again to recheck the PEEK prosthesis's accurate position, known as the third navigation or "Simulation-Guided Navigation" (SGN).

Accuracy was postoperatively verified by superimposing the postoperative CT scan onto the preoperative CT scan, which contained the surgical plan. Measurements were then taken in the axial, sagittal, and coronal planes.

This study was conducted in accordance with the tenets of the WMA Declaration of Helsinki in the context of Ethical Principles for Medical Research Involving Human Subjects. It was approved by our institution's local institutional review board (Act. number 301, ref. 4626; 03-2020).

3. Results

The study sample comprised three females and one male, with an average age of 47.5 years old. One lesion was in the supraorbital rim and orbital roof, one in the frontal bone and orbital roof and two in the zygomatic region (Table 1). CANPS was successfully performed.

There were no complications related to navigated surgery. The surgery could be performed according to the surgical plan with a precision of 1 mm.

The use of the navigated piezoelectric device reduced the surgeon's uncertainty during the osteotomies in depth and in poorly visible areas. Three experienced surgeons, two maxillofacial surgeons and one plastic surgeon with experience in facial reconstruction, independently assessed the esthetic result as excellent in all four patients. The evaluation was performed using a five-choice graded scale: poor, fair, satisfactory, very satisfactory and excellent. Figures 1–9 represent Case 2. Figures 10–18 illustrate Case 3.

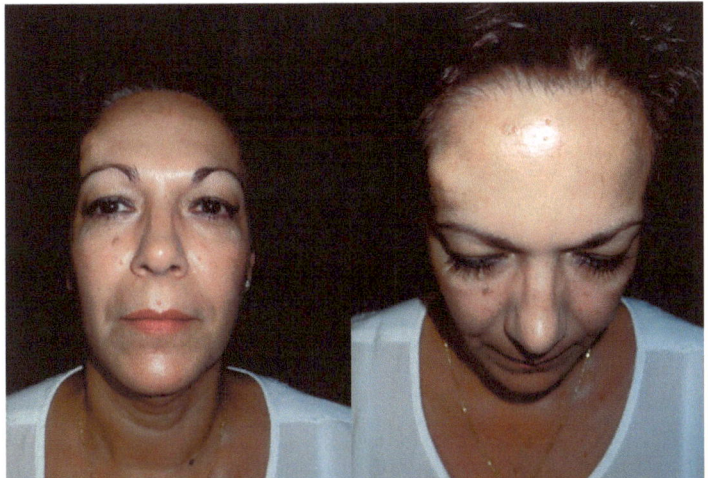

Figure 1. These images show the preoperative external appearance of the face of Patient 2. The protrusion can be seen in the right frontal region due to an intraosseous venous malformation.

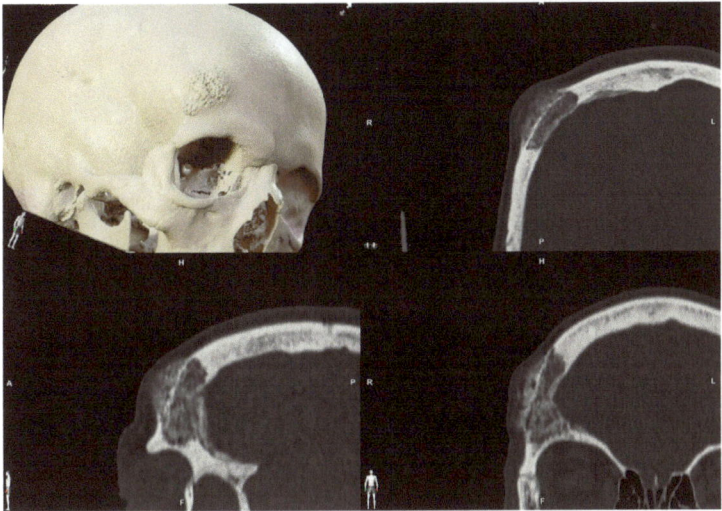

Figure 2. Preoperative CT scan. Three-dimensional, axial, sagittal and coronal views can be appreciated. There is a mixed radiolucent lesion and an expansive lytic defect affecting the frontal bone above the right supraorbital rim and roof of the right orbit. A: anterior, P: posterior, H: head, F: foot, R: right, L: left.

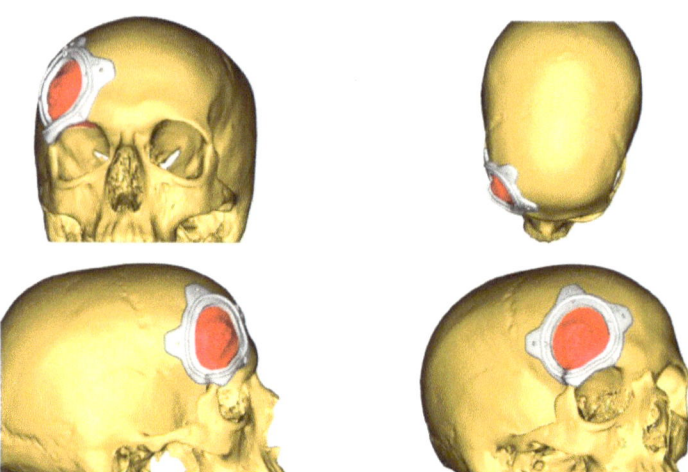

Figure 3. The resection plan (in red in the figure) and the surgical cutting guide that will conduct the resection on the surface of the frontal bone as planned.

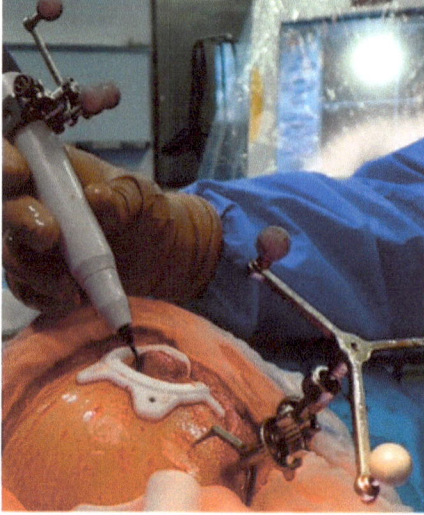

Figure 4. Navigated piezoelectric device. Direct or "live" navigation of the frontal bone. The skull post was anchored with a self-drilling screw.

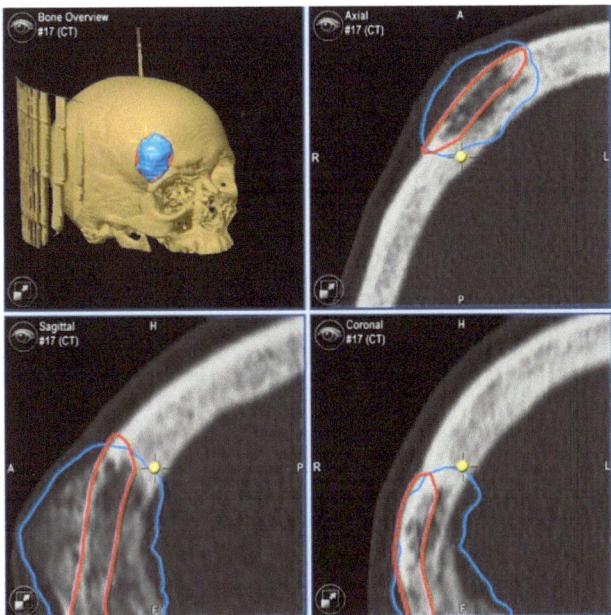

Figure 5. Images of direct navigation with the piezoelectric device (yellow dot with small cross) are shown on the navigation screen. The progression and depth of the guided osteotomy can be appreciated and evaluated in real time ("live navigation"). A: anterior, P: posterior, H: head, F: foot, R: right, L: left. In blue, the virtual resection; in red, the virtual reconstruction with the PEEK prosthesis.

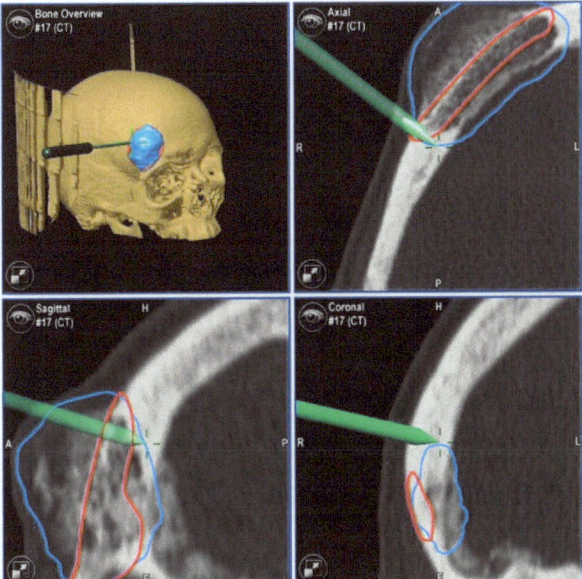

Figure 6. With the navigation pointer, the osteotomy (indirect navigation) we perform (green line on the navigation screen) can also be checked. A: anterior, P: posterior, H: head, F: foot, R: right, L: left. In blue, the virtual resection; in red, the virtual reconstruction with the PEEK prosthesis.

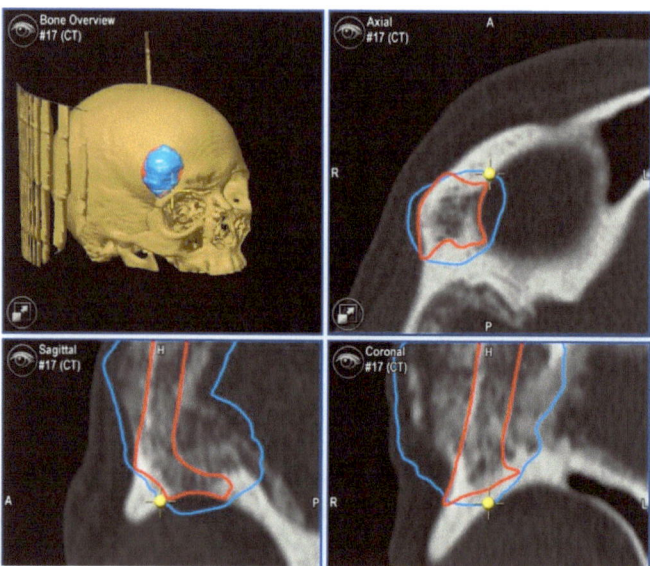

Figure 7. Images of direct navigation of the right orbital roof with the navigated piezoelectric device (yellow dot with small cross) are shown on the navigation screen. The progression and depth of the guided osteotomy can be appreciated and evaluated in real time ("live navigation"). A: anterior, P: posterior, H: head, F: foot, R: right, L: left. In blue, the virtual resection; in red, the virtual reconstruction with the PEEK prosthesis.

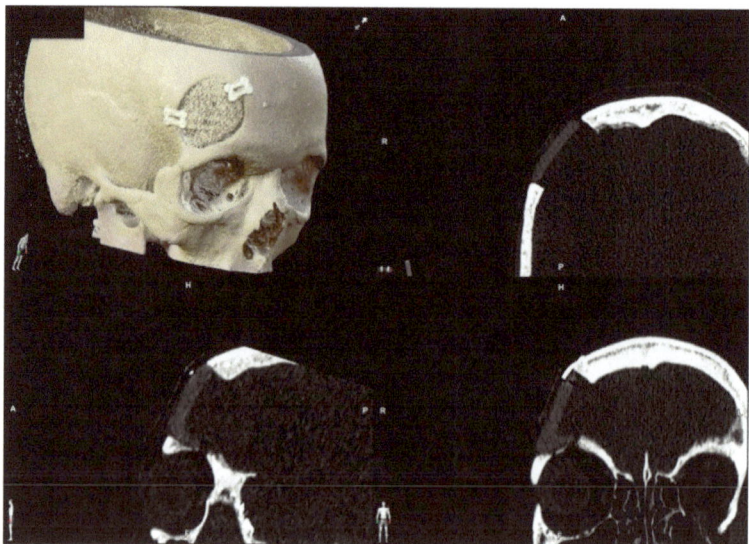

Figure 8. Postoperative CT scan. Three-dimensional, axial, sagittal and coronal views can be appreciated.

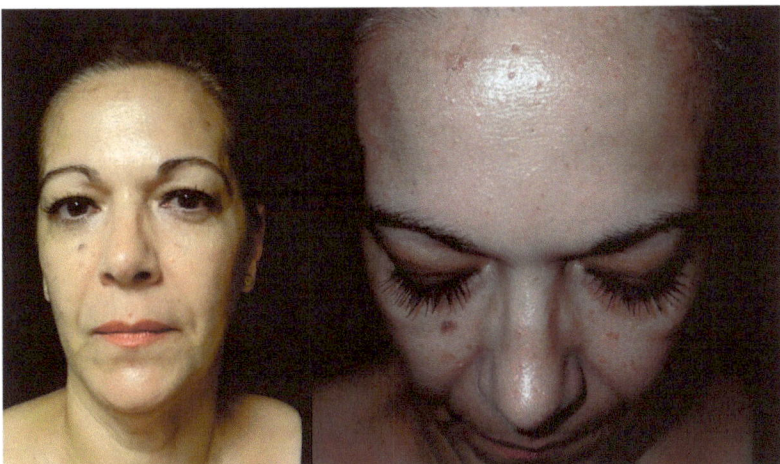

Figure 9. These images show the postoperative facial appearance with reestablishment of the frontal contour.

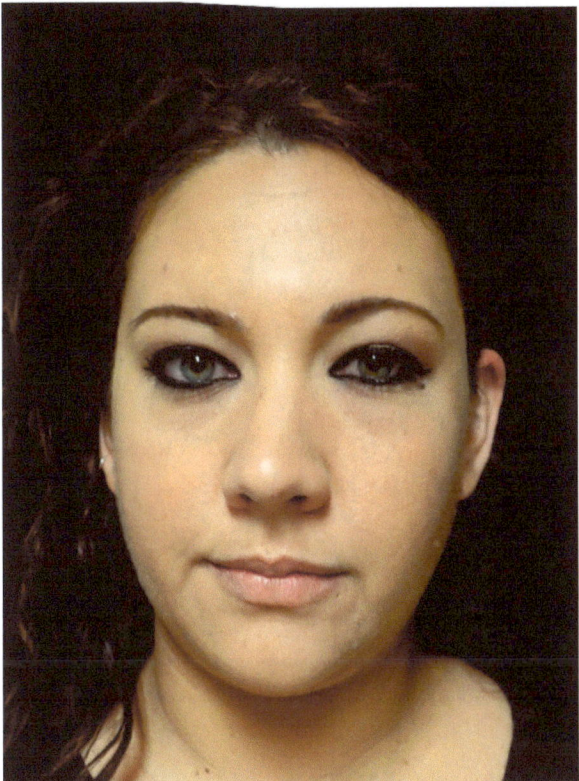

Figure 10. This image shows the preoperative external appearance of the face of Patient 3. There is a slight elevation of the left eyeball and a protrusion of the left cheek.

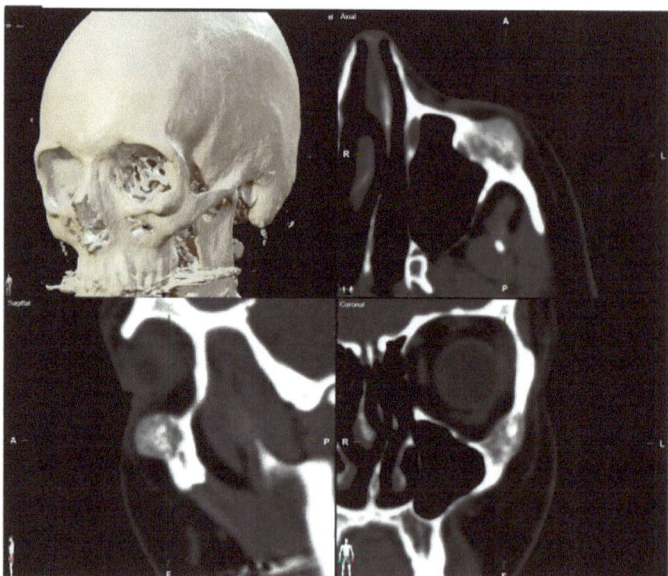

Figure 11. Preoperative CT scan. Three-dimensional, axial, sagittal and coronal views can be appreciated. There are a mixed radiolucent lesion and an expansive lytic defect affecting the left infraorbital rim, zygoma, external zone of the orbital floor and inferior part of the external wall.

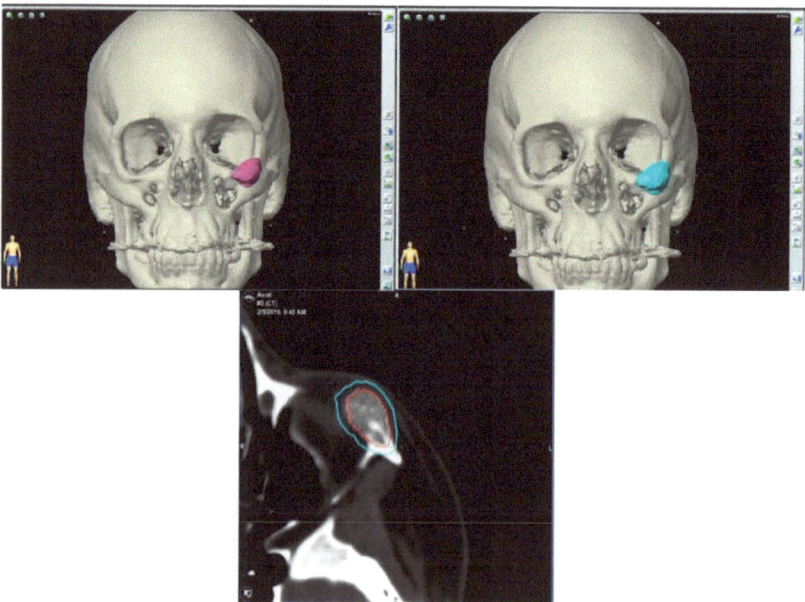

Figure 12. Surgical plan with the BrainLab® navigation software, iPlan® 3.0.6 (Munich, Germany). The lesion is colored in red and the surgical margin in blue.

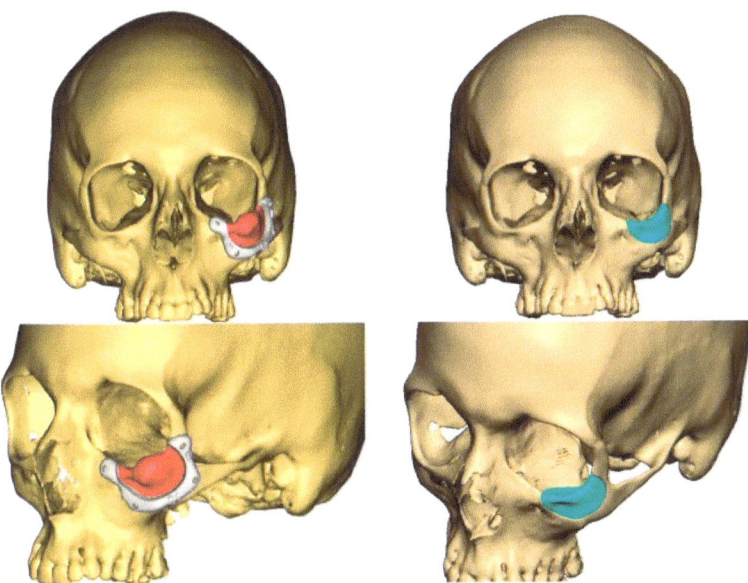

Figure 13. This image shows the lesion (in red), the surgical guide (in white) and the planned PEEK prosthesis (in blue).

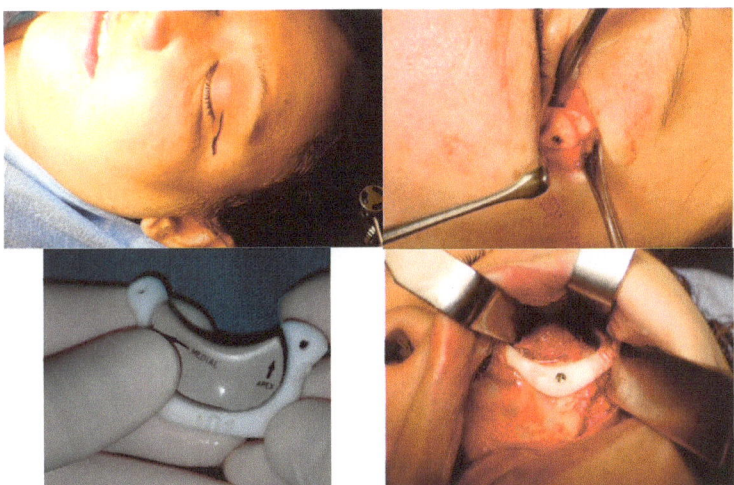

Figure 14. This picture shows the surgical approach to the orbit, the surgical guide and the prosthesis, the vestibular intraoral approach with the surgical guide in position anchored to the zygoma with screws and the superior osteotomy line.

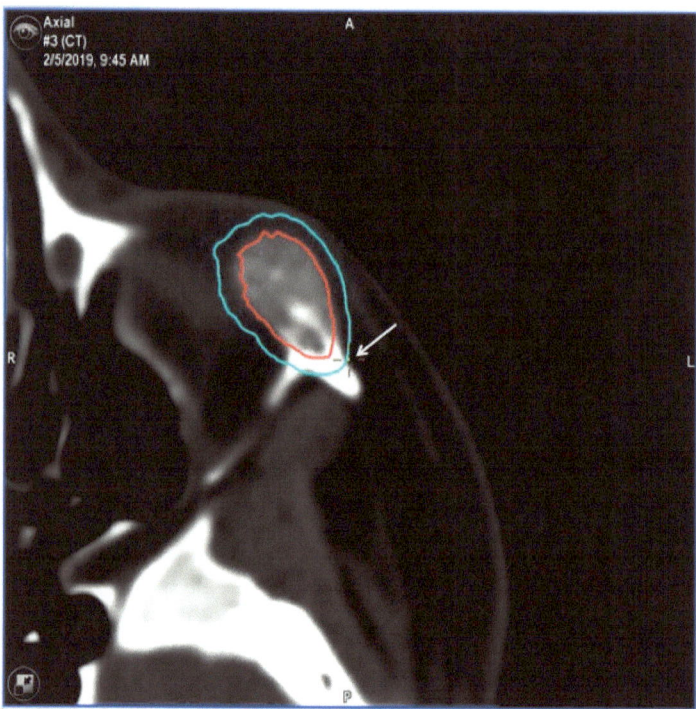

Figure 15. Images of direct navigation with the piezoelectric device on the less-visible posterior part the zygoma (yellow dot with small cross) are shown on the navigation screen. Again, the progression and depth of the guided osteotomy can be appreciated and evaluated in real time ("live navigation"). The lesion is colored in red and the surgical margin in blue.

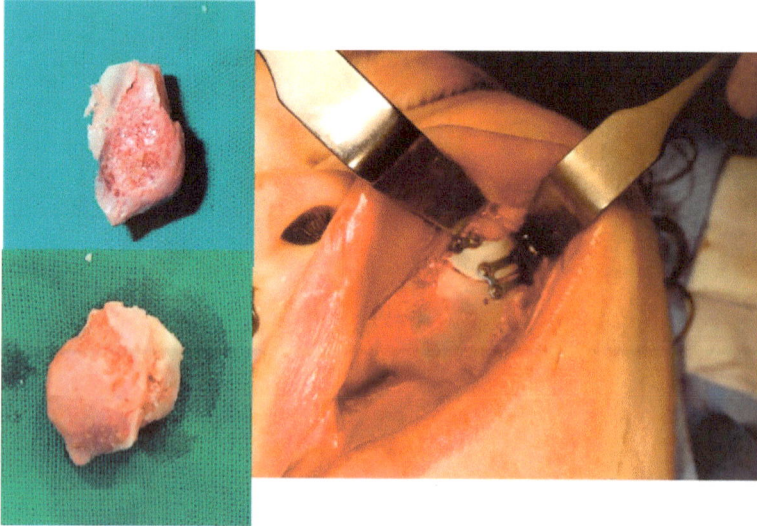

Figure 16. The resected lesion, the PEEK prosthesis and the osteosynthesis with miniplates (intraoral approach).

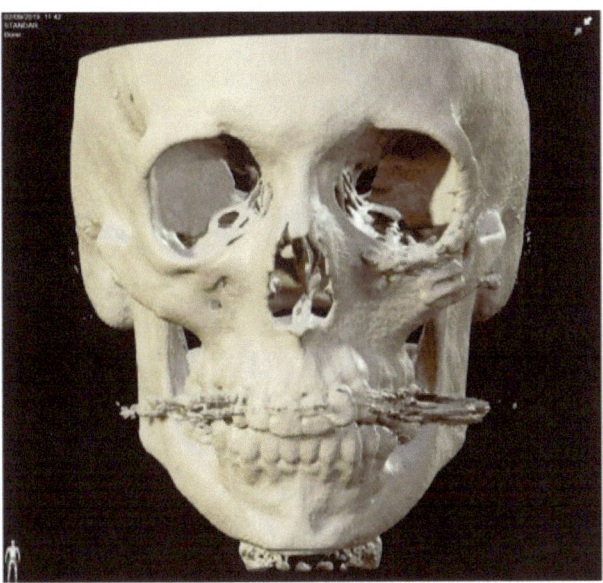

Figure 17. Postoperative 3D CT.

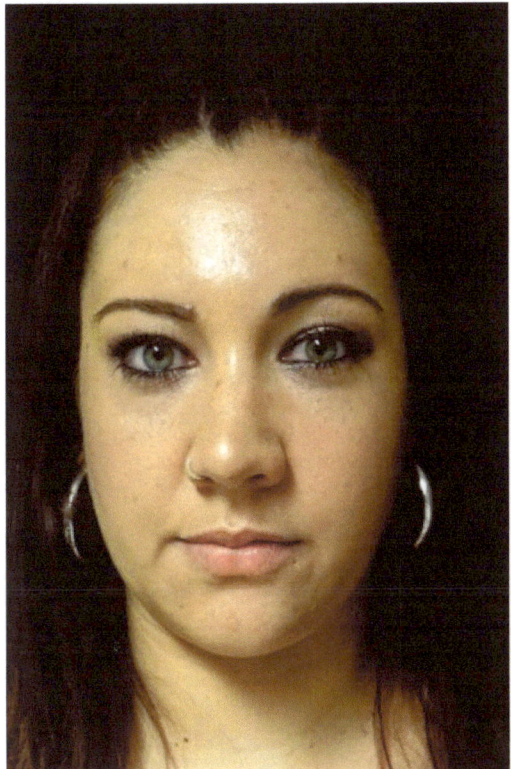

Figure 18. Postoperative facial appearance.

4. Discussion

The use of virtual surgical planning, CAD-CAM design of prostheses and customized surgical guides has been applied by a few authors for the surgical management of vascular anomalies of the facial bones [9,41,51,52]. To the best of our knowledge, no paper has combined surgical navigation with these technologies. Moreover, it is also the first time that both indirect surgical navigation with a pointer and direct surgical navigation with the piezoelectric device have been performed to resect vascular anomalies of facial bones.

Intraosseous vascular anomalies of the facial skeleton represent a diagnostic and therapeutic challenge for craniofacial surgeons. Computer-assisted technology for virtual planning, CAD-CAM designed PEEK prosthesis, surgical navigation and piezoelectric resection represent a new trend in the multidisciplinary treatment of these complex anomalies. This technology improves cutting precision and intraoperative safety, helping to minimize esthetically impairing scars and surgical morbidity, achieving exceptional outcomes in this anatomical region.

Careful clinical and radiographic evaluation is essential to avoid misdiagnosing hemangiomas, venous malformations, and arteriovenous malformations. Histopathological and immunohistochemical analyses may be required in some cases.

We, as many authors, recommend immediate reconstruction after surgical resection. Common reconstructive options include autogenous calvarial graft [27,53,54], pre-bent titanium mesh on a standard or a patient stereolithographic model [19,55], and customized PEEK (Polyetheretheretherketone), titanium, methyl-methacrylate prostheses or polycaprolactone/beta tricalcium phosphate scaffold [9,12,51,52,56–62]. Customized prostheses allow for a reliable reconstruction with excellent esthetic results, avoid morbidity in the donor site, and reduce surgical time.

When comparing reconstruction materials, PEEK has similar strength and weight to human bone, offers high biocompatibility and durability, is radiolucent and has low rates of infection and allergic reactions, but can be expensive and has a higher infection rate compared to titanium. Titanium prostheses are strong, biocompatible and have superior osseointegration potential, but are radiopaque, expensive and difficult to modify during surgery. Both PEEK and titanium can be sterilized and customized. PEEK mimics bone elasticity and density better, is adjustable during surgery, and can increase in thickness to restore volume, but requires titanium screws for fixation due to its poor osseointegration. Autologous bone grafts integrate well biologically with minimal rejection, but may cause donor site morbidity and are in limited availability. PMMA is a cost-effective and easy to shape bone cement, but presents a higher risk of infection, especially for long-term use [60–62].

Several authors have reported that the use of virtual surgery and CAD-CAM design of prostheses and customized surgical guides improves the accuracy of the reconstruction and its esthetic results, reduces complications of ablation and reconstruction, and decreases surgical time and postoperative hospital stay [12,51,57]. In our cases, we could establish that there was less than 1 mm of difference between the planned resection and reconstruction with the postoperative CTs. The esthetic results were excellent in all cases according to the surgeon's and patients' appreciation. Shorter surgeries minimize the risk of infection and other intraoperative complications, while shorter hospital stays benefit patient recovery. From our point of view, the integration of virtual surgery, CAD-CAM design and surgical navigation technology represents a significant advancement in reconstructive surgery [42–47,59].

According to the two types of navigation methods, "indirect" or "sequential" navigation uses a probe intermittently. In contrast, "direct", live, continuous, or real-time navigation" registers the operating instrument as a probe, allowing for continuous navigation during surgery. CANPS is a "direct" navigation [49,50]. CANPS can be applied to guide osteotomies in depth and in areas where it is impossible to place surgical guides because of their limited accessibility. CANPS can be used to control these hidden osteotomies during the resection of facial intraosseous vascular malformations [48,49]. Navigation can be once more used to verify the precise placement of the PEEK prosthesis, a process referred to as the third navigation or "Simulation-Guided Navigation" (SGN).

The advantages of computer planning and surgical navigation in treating intraosseous vascular malformations include accurate preoperative diagnosis, virtual surgery simulation, improved reconstruction accuracy, increased surgical safety, "direct navigation" or real-time guidance during surgery, reducing the risk of injury to anatomical structures, and operative time. The use of the navigation systems saves overall surgical time by decreasing uncertainty and increasing the surgeon's confidence and precision with the resection and the reconstruction [41,43,45–47,59].

Possible complications related to virtual planning and surgical navigation are as follows: errors in planning and establishing appropriate surgical resection margins, loss of accuracy during surgical navigation, loosening of the screw that fixes the skull post with the dynamic reference frame to the skull, and inadvertent injuries with the navigation instruments.

We describe a novel surgical strategy for facial intraosseous vascular anomalies, using minimally invasive resection with piezosurgery and surgical navigation. It provides precise and confident resection and reconstruction but has an initial cost and learning curve drawbacks. Navigation saves time by decreasing uncertainty but requires preoperative planning and takes up space in the operating room.

5. Conclusions

Resection of facial intraosseous vascular anomalies can benefit from using CAD-CAM technologies, Computer-assisted navigated piezoelectric surgery and surgical navigation. CAD-CAM allows for the manufacture of PEEK prostheses that can be immediately adapted to the defect. Surgical navigation allows for the performance of osteotomies according to the planning, maximizing surgical precision and safety.

Author Contributions: Conceptualization, A.D. and F.J.A.; methodology, A.D. and F.J.A.; software, A.D., O.E. and F.J.A.; validation, A.D., O.E., C.C., A.S.-S., M.E.S.-F. and F.J.A.; formal analysis, A.D., O.E., C.C., A.S.-S., M.E.S.-F. and F.J.A.; investigation, A.D. and F.J.A.; resources, A.D., O.E., C.C., A.S.-S., M.E.S.-F. and F.J.A.; data curation, A.D. and F.J.A.; writing—original draft preparation, A.D., A.S.-S. and F.J.A.; writing—review and editing, A.D., O.E., C.C., A.S.-S., M.E.S.-F. and F.J.A.; visualization, A.D.; supervision, F.J.A.; project administration, A.D. All authors have read and agreed to the published version of the manuscript.

Funding: This research received no external funding.

Institutional Review Board Statement: This study was conducted in accordance with the Declaration of Helsinki, and approved by the Institutional Review Board (or Ethics Committee) of HOSPITAL UNIVERSITARIO REINA SOFÍA. CÓRDOBA. SPAIN (Act. number 301, ref. 4626; 03-2020).

Informed Consent Statement: Informed consent was obtained from all subjects involved in the study. Written informed consent was obtained from the patient(s) to publish this paper.

Data Availability Statement: The data presented in this study are available on request from the corresponding authors.

Acknowledgments: We would like to thank all members of the Maxillofacial and Neurosurgery Department of the University Hospital Reina Sofía, Córdoba, Spain.

Conflicts of Interest: The authors declare no conflicts of interest.

References

1. Liberale, C.; Rozell-Shannon, L.; Moneghini, L.; Nocini, R.; Tombris, S.; Colletti, G. Stop calling me cavernous hemangioma! A literature review on misdiagnosed bony vascular anomalies. *J. Investig. Surg.* **2022**, *15*, 141–150. [CrossRef] [PubMed]
2. Mulliken, J.B.; Glowacki, J.; Mulliken, J.B.; Glowacki, J. Hemangiomas and vascular malformations in infants and children: A classification based on endothelial characteristics. *Plast. Reconstr. Surg.* **1982**, *69*, 412–422. [CrossRef] [PubMed]
3. Behr, G.G.; Johnson, C.J. Vascular anomalies: Hemangiomas and beyond- Part I, fast-flow lesions. *Am. J. Roentgenol. AJR* **2013**, *200*, 414–422. [CrossRef]

4. Wassef, M.; Blei, F.; Adams, D.; Alomari, A.; Baselga, E.; Berestein, A.; Burrows, P.; Frieden, I.J.; Garzon, M.C.; Lopez-Gutierrez, J.C.; et al. Vascular anomalies classification: Recommendations from the international society for the study of vascular anomalies. *Pediatrics* **2015**, *136*, e203–e214. [CrossRef]
5. Kadlub, N.; Dainese, L.; Coulomb-L'Hermine, A.; Galmiche, L.; Soupre, V.; Ducou Lepointe, H.; Vazquez, M.P.; Picard, A. Intraosseous haemangioma: Semantic and medical confusion. *Int. J. Oral Maxillofac. Surg.* **2015**, *44*, 718–724. [CrossRef]
6. Defazio, M.V.; Kassira, W.; Camison, L.; Meshkov, L.; Robinson, P.G.; Kawamoto, H.K.; Thaller, S.R. Intraosseous venous malformations of the zygoma: Clarification of misconceptions regarding diagnosis and management. *Ann. Plast. Surg.* **2014**, *72*, 323–327. [CrossRef] [PubMed]
7. Colletti, G.; Frigerio, A.; Giovanditto, F.; Biglioli, F.; Chiapasco, M.; Grimmer, J. Surgical treatment of vascular malformations of the facial bones. *J. Oral Maxillofac. Surg.* **2014**, *72*, 1326.e1–1326.e18. [CrossRef]
8. Valentini, V.; Nicolai, G.; Loré, B.; Aboh, I.V. Intraosseous hemangiomas. *J. Craniofac. Surg.* **2008**, *19*, 1459–1464. [CrossRef] [PubMed]
9. Powers, D.B.; Fisher, E.; Erdmann, D. Zygomatic Intraosseous Hemangioma: Case Report and Literature Review. *Craniomaxillofac. Trauma Reconstr.* **2017**, *10*, 1–10. [CrossRef]
10. Yu, M.S.; Kim, H.C.; Jang, Y.J. Removal of a nasal bone intraosseous venous malformation and primary reconstruction of the surgical defect using open rhinoplasty. *Int. J. Oral Maxillofac. Surg.* **2010**, *39*, 394–396. [CrossRef]
11. Park, B.H.; Hwang, E.; Kim, C.H. Primary intraosseous hemangioma in the frontal bone. *Arch. Plast. Surg.* **2013**, *40*, 283–285. [CrossRef] [PubMed]
12. Brandner, J.S.; Rawal, Y.B.; Kim, L.J.; Dillon, J.K. Intraosseous Hemangioma of the Frontal Bone. Report of a Case and Review of the Literature. *J. Oral Maxillofac. Surg.* **2018**, *76*, 799–805. [CrossRef] [PubMed]
13. Sweet, C.; Silbergleit, R.; Mehta, B. Primary intraosseous hemangioma of the orbit: CT and MR appearance. *Am. J. Neuroradiol.* **1997**, *18*, 379–381. [PubMed]
14. Marshak, G. Hemangioma of the zygomatic bone. *Arch. Otolaryngol.* **1980**, *106*, 581–582. [CrossRef] [PubMed]
15. Moore, S.L.; Chun, J.K.; Mitre, S.A.; Som, P.M. Intraosseous hemangioma of the zygoma: CT and MR findings. *Am. J. Neuroradiol.* **2001**, *22*, 1383–1385. [PubMed]
16. Zucker, J.J.; Levine, M.R.; Chu, A. Primary intraosseous hemangioma of the orbit. Report of a case and review of literature. *Ophthal Plast. Reconstr. Surg.* **1989**, *5*, 247–255. [CrossRef]
17. Relf, S.J.; Bartley, G.B.; Unni, K.K. Primary orbital intraosseous hemangioma. *Ophthalmology* **1991**, *98*, 541–546. [CrossRef]
18. Cheng, N.C.; Lai, D.M.; Hsie, M.H.; Liao, S.L.; Chen, Y.B. Intraosseous hemangiomas of the facial bone. *Plast. Reconstr. Surg.* **2006**, *117*, 2366–2372. [CrossRef]
19. Temerek, A.T.; Ali, S.; Shehab, M.F. Computer guided resection and reconstruction of intra-osseous zygomatic hemangioma: Case report and systematic review of literature. *Int. J. Surg. Case Rep.* **2020**, *66*, 240–256. [CrossRef]
20. Taylan, G.; Yildirim, S.; Gideroğlu, K.; Aköz, T. Conservative approach in a rare case of intrazygomatic hemangioma. *Plast. Reconstr. Surg.* **2003**, *112*, 1490–1492. [CrossRef]
21. Dereci, O.; Acikalin, M.F.; Ay, S. Unusual intraosseous capillary hemangioma of the mandible. *Eur. J. Dent.* **2015**, *9*, 438–441. [CrossRef] [PubMed]
22. Gologorsky, Y.; Shivastava, R.K.; Panov, F.; Mascitelli, J.; Del Signore, A.; Govindarajj, S.; Smethurst, M.; Bronster, D.J. Primary intraosseous cavernous hemangioma of the clivus: Case report and review of the literature. *J. Neurol. Surg. Rep.* **2013**, *74*, 17–22. [CrossRef] [PubMed]
23. Hirai, S.; Saigusa, K. Intraosseous cystic cavernous angioma with occipital skull osteolysis. *Interdiscip. Neurosurg. Adv. Tech. Case Manag.* **2014**, *1*, 53–55. [CrossRef]
24. Perugini, M.; Renzi, G.; Gasparini, G.; Cerulli, G.; Becelli, R. Intraosseous hemangioma of the maxillofacial district: Clinical analysisi and surgical treatment in 10 consecutive patients. *J. Craniofac. Surg.* **2004**, *15*, 980–985. [CrossRef] [PubMed]
25. Gonçalves, F.G.; Ovalle-Rojas, J.P.; Hanagandi, P.B.; Valente, R.; Torres, C.I.; Chankwosky, J.; DelCardio-O'Donovan, R. Case report: Periorbital intraosseous hemanggiomas. *Indian J. Radiol. Imaging* **2011**, *21*, 287–291. [CrossRef] [PubMed]
26. Myadam, V.; Kishan, V.; Deepa, A.; Puja, K.S.; Rani, K.D. Intraosseous hemangioma of the zygomatic bone: A rare site for hemangioma. *Med. J. Armed Forces India* **2016**, *72*, 85–87. [CrossRef] [PubMed]
27. Cuesta Gil, M.; Navarro-Vila, C. Intraosseous hemangioma of the zygomatic bone. A case report. *Int. J. Oral Maxillofac. Surg.* **1992**, *21*, 287–291. [CrossRef] [PubMed]
28. Torrres-Carranza, A.; García-Perla, A.; Infante-Cossío, P.; Acosta-Feria, M.; Belmonte-Caro, R.; Gutiérrez-Pérez, J.L. Hemangioma intraóseo primario de la órbita: A propósito de dos casos. *Neurocirugía* **2007**, *18*, 320–325. [CrossRef]
29. Magde, S.N.; Simon, S.; Abidin, Z.; Ghabrial, R.; Davis, G.; McNab, A.; Selva, D. Primary orbital intraosseous hemangioma. *Ophthal Plast. Reconstr. Surg.* **2009**, *25*, 37–41.
30. Marcinow, A.M.; Provenzano, M.J.; Gurgel, R.K.; Chang, K.E. Primary intraosseous cavernous hemangioma of the zygoma: A case report and literature review. *Ear Nose Throat J.* **2012**, *91*, 210–215. [CrossRef]
31. Choi, J.S.; Bae, Y.C.; Kang, G.B.; Choi, K.U. Intraosseous hemangioma of the orbit. *Arch. Craniofac. Surg.* **2018**, *19*, 68–71. [CrossRef] [PubMed]
32. Akther, A.; El Tecle, N.; Alexopoulos, G.; Espinoza, G.; Coppens, J. Intraosseous Orbital Cavernous Hemangioma with Frontal Extension and Dural Involvement. *Cureus* **2019**, *11*, e4823. [CrossRef]

33. Salvador, E.; Hilario-Barrio, A.; Martín-Medina, P.; Koren-Fernandez, L.; Ramos-Gonzalez, A.; Martinez de Aragón, A. Facial Intraosseous Haemangioma. *Eurorad* **2019**, Case 16421. [CrossRef]
34. Colletti, G.; Lerardi, A.M. Understanding venous malformations of the head and neck: A comprehensive insight. *Med. Oncol.* **2017**, *34*, 42. [CrossRef]
35. Fernández, L.R.; Luberti, R.; Dominguez, F.V. Aspectos radiográficos de los hemangiomas óseos maxilo-faciales. Revisión bibliográfica y presentación de dos casos. *Med. Oral* **2003**, *8*, 166–177.
36. Koybasi, S.; Saydam, L.; Kutluay, L. Intraosseous hemangioma of the zygoma. *Am. J. Otolaryngol.* **2003**, *24*, 194–197. [CrossRef] [PubMed]
37. Zhu, C.; Zhu, H.G.; Zhang, Z.Y.; Wang, L.Z.; Zheng, J.W.; Ye, W.M.; He, Y.; Wang, Y.A. Intraosseous venous malformations of the facial bone: A retrospective study in 11 patients. *Phlebology* **2013**, *28*, 257–263. [CrossRef]
38. Taschner, C.A.; Brendeeke, S.; Campos, M.; Urbach, H.; Lützen, N.; Prinz, M. Freiburg Neuropathology case conference: Periorbital bone lesion causing proptosis in a 31-year-old patient. *Clin. Neuroradiol.* **2014**, *24*, 399–403. [CrossRef]
39. Seeff, J.; Blacksin, M.F.; Lyons, M.; Benevenia, J. A case report of intracortical hemangioma. A forgotten intracortical lesion. *Clin. Orthop. Relat. Res.* **1994**, *302*, 235–238. [CrossRef]
40. Park, S.-M.; Lee, J.-H. Recurrence of intraosseous cavernous hemangioma in the maxilla: A case report. *Oral Maxillofac. Surg. Cases* **2020**, *6*, 100147. [CrossRef]
41. Azarmehr, I.; Stokbro, K.; Bell, R.B.; Thygesen, T. Surgical navigation: A systematic review of indications, treatments, and outcomes in oral and maxillofacial surgery. *J. Oral Maxillofac. Surg.* **2017**, *75*, 1987–2005. [CrossRef] [PubMed]
42. Schramm, A.; Suárez-Cunqueiro, M.M.; Barth, E.L.; Essig, H.; Bormann, K.H.; Kokemueller, H.; Rücker, M.; Gellrich, N.C. Computer-Assisted Navigation in craniomaxillofacial tumors. *J. Craniofac. Surg.* **2008**, *19*, 1067–1074. [CrossRef]
43. Schramm, A.; Suarez-Cunqueiro, M.M.; Rücker, M.; Kokemueller, H.; Bormann, K.H.; Metzger, M.C.; Gellrich, N.C. Computer-assisted therapy in orbital and mid-facial reconstructions. *Int. J. Med. Robot. Comput. Assist. Surg.* **2009**, *5*, 111–124. [CrossRef]
44. Heiland, M.; Habermann, C.R.; Schmelzle, R. Indications and limitations of intraoperative navigation in maxillofacial surgery. *J. Oral Maxillofac. Surg.* **2004**, *62*, 1059–1063. [CrossRef]
45. Rana, M.; Essig, H.; Eckardt, A.M.; Tavassol, F.; Ruecker, M.; Schramm, A.; Gellrich, N.C. Advances and innovations in Computer-Assisted head and neck oncologic surgery. *J. Craniofac. Surg.* **2012**, *23*, 272–278. [CrossRef]
46. Markiewicz, M.R.; Dierks, E.J.; Bell, R.B. Does intraoperative navigation restore orbital dimensions in traumatic and post-ablative defects? *J. Cranio-Maxillofac. Surg.* **2012**, *40*, 142–148. [CrossRef] [PubMed]
47. Yu, H.; Shen, S.G.; Wang, X.; Zhang, L.; Zhang, S. The indication and application of computer-assisted navigation in oral and maxillofacial surgery- Shanghai's experience based on 104 cases. *J. Craniomaxillofac. Surg.* **2013**, *41*, 770–774. [CrossRef]
48. Bianchi, A.; Badiali, G.; Piersanti, L.; Marchetti, C. Computer-Assisted Piezoelectric Surgery: A navigated approach toward performance of craniomaxillofacial osteotomies. *J. Craniofac. Surg.* **2015**, *26*, 867–872. [CrossRef]
49. Dean, A.; Heredero, S.; Solivera, J.; Sanjuan, A.; Alamillos, F.J. Computer-assisted and navigated piezoelectric surgery: A new technology to improve precision and surgical safety in craniomaxillofacial surgery. *Laryngoscope Investig. Otolaryngol.* **2022**, *7*, 684–691. [CrossRef]
50. Dean, A.; Alamillos, F.J.; Heredero, S.; Solivera, J. A novel technique to secure the skull post in a thin skull allowing for surgical navigation in infants. *J. Oral Maxillofac. Surg.* **2020**, *78*, 284.e1–284.e4. [CrossRef]
51. Antúnez-Conde, R.; Navarro-Cuellar, C.; Salmerón-Escobar, J.I.; Díez-Montiel, A.; Navarro-Cuellar, I.; Dell'Aversana-Orabona, G.; Del Castillo-Pardo de Vera, J.L.; Navarro-Vila, C.; Cebrián-Carretero, J.L. Intraosseous venous malformation of the zygomatic bone: Comparison between virtual surgical planning and standard surgery with review of the literature. *J. Clin. Med.* **2021**, *10*, 4565. [CrossRef] [PubMed]
52. Rios-Vicil, C.I.; Barbery, D.; Dang, P.; Jean, W.C. Single-stage cranioplasty with customized polyetheretherketone implant after tumor resection using virtual reality and augmented reality for precise implant customization and placement: Illustrative case. *J. Neurosurg. Case Lessons* **2022**, *3*, 2255. [CrossRef]
53. Pinna, V.; Clauser, L.; Marchi, M.; Castellan, L. Haemangioma of the zygoma: Case report. *Neuroradiology* **1997**, *39*, 216–218. [CrossRef] [PubMed]
54. Zins, J.E.; Türegün, M.C.; Hosn, W.; Bauer, T.W. Reconstruction of intraosseous hemangiomas of the midface using split calvarial bone grafts. *Plast. Reconstr. Surg.* **2006**, *117*, 948–953. [CrossRef]
55. Bocchialini, G.; Castellani, A.; Bozzola, A.; Rossi, A. A Hemangioma of the Zygomatic Bone: Management Ensuring Good Reconstructive and Aesthetic Results. *Craniomaxillofac. Trauma Reconstr.* **2017**, *10*, 332–336. [CrossRef] [PubMed]
56. Arribas-Garcia, I.; Alcala-Galiano, A.; Fernandez Garcia, A.; Montalvo, J.J. Zygomatic intraosseous haemangioma: Reconstruction with an alloplastic prosthesis based on a 3-D model. *J. Plast. Reconstr. Aesthet. Surg.* **2010**, *63*, e451–e453. [CrossRef] [PubMed]
57. Yashin, K.S.; Ermolaev, A.Y.; Ostapyuk, M.V.; Kutlaeva, M.A.; Rasteryaeva, M.V.; Mlyaykh, S.G.; Medyanik, I.A. Case report: Simultaneous resection of bone tumor and CAD/CAM titanium cranioplasty in fronto-orbital region. *Front. Surg.* **2018**, *8*, 718725. [CrossRef]
58. Jeong, W.S.; Kim, Y.C.; Min, J.C.; Park, H.J.; Lee, E.J.; Shim, J.H.; Choi, J.W. Clinical application of 3D-printed patient-specific polycaprolactone/beta tricalcicum phosphate scaffold for complex zygomatico-maxillary defects. *Polymers* **2022**, *14*, 740. [CrossRef] [PubMed]

59. Metzger, M.C.; Hohlweg-Majert, B.; Schön, R.; Teschner, M.; Gellrich, N.C.; Schmelzeisen, R.; Gutwald, R. Verification of clinical precision after computer-aided reconstruction in craniomaxillofacial surgery. *Oral Surg. Oral Med. Oral Pathol. Oral Radiol. Endod.* **2007**, *104*, e1–e10. [CrossRef]
60. Gerbino, G.; Zavatero, E.; Zenga, F.; Bianchi, F.A.; Garnizo-Demo, P.; Berrone, S. Primary and secondary reconstruction of complex craniofacial defects using polyetherketone custom-made implants. *J. Craniomaxillofac.* **2015**, *43*, 1356–1363. [CrossRef]
61. Cárdenas-Serres, C.; Almeida-Parra, F.; Simón-Flors, A.M.; de Leyva-Moreno, P.; Ranz-Colio, Á.; Ley-Urzaiz, L.; Acero-Sanz, J. Custom CAD/CAM Peek Implants for complex orbitocranial reconstruction: Our experience with 15 patients. *J. Clin. Med.* **2024**, *13*, 695. [CrossRef] [PubMed]
62. Kim, M.M.; Boahene, K.D.O.; Byrne, P.J. Use of Customized Polyetheretherketone (PEEK) Implants in the Reconstruction of Complex Maxillofacial Defects. *Arch. Fac. Plast. Surg.* **2009**, *11*, 53–57. [CrossRef] [PubMed]

Disclaimer/Publisher's Note: The statements, opinions and data contained in all publications are solely those of the individual author(s) and contributor(s) and not of MDPI and/or the editor(s). MDPI and/or the editor(s) disclaim responsibility for any injury to people or property resulting from any ideas, methods, instructions or products referred to in the content.

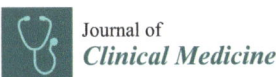

Article

Long-Term Functional Outcomes Following Enzymatic Debridement of Deep Hand Burns Using Nexobrid®: A Retrospective Analysis

Asja T. Malsagova [1,*], Amin El-Habbassi [2], Moritz Billner [1], Maresa Berns [1], Tamas Pueski [1], Karl J. Bodenschatz [3], Paul I. Heidekrueger [4,†] and Denis Ehrl [1,†]

1. Department for Plastic, Reconstructive and Hand Surgery, Burn Center for Severe Burn Injuries, Nuremberg Hospital, Paracelsus Medical University, Breslauer Str. 201, 90471 Nuremberg/Prof.-Ernst-Nathan Straße 1, 90419 Nuremberg, Germany; moritz.billner@klinikum-nuernberg.de (M.B.); maresa.berns@klinikum-nuernberg.de (M.B.); tamas.pueski@klinikum-nuernberg.de (T.P.); denis.ehrl@klinikum-nuernberg.de (D.E.)
2. Paracelsus Medical University Salzburg, Muellner Hauptstr. 48, 5020 Salzburg, Austria; amin.habbassi@stud.pmu.ac.at
3. Department for Pediatric Surgery, Nuremberg Hospital, Paracelsus Medical University, Breslauer Str. 201, 90471 Nuremberg/Prof.-Ernst-Nathan Straße 1, 90419 Nuremberg, Germany; karl.bodenschatz@klinikum-nuernberg.de
4. Centre of Plastic, Aesthetic, Hand and Reconstructive Surgery, University of Regensburg, Universitätsstraße 31, 93053 Regensburg, Germany; paul@heidekrueger.net
* Correspondence: asja.malsagova@gmail.com
† These authors contributed equally to this work.

Abstract: Background: For years, surgical debridement with autografting has been considered the standard of care in the treatment of severe burns of the hand. However, in recent years, enzymatic debridement has increasingly been reported as a good alternative, especially for burns of the hand, as it selectively preserves viable tissue. In this study, we aim to evaluate the long-term function of the hand after enzymatic debridement in deep dermal burns. **Methods**: A retrospective chart review was conducted as well as measurements of subjective and objective outcome measures through physical examination and Disabilities of the Arm, Shoulder, and Hand (DASH), Patient and Observer Scar Assessment Scale (POSAS), and Vancouver Scar Scale (VSS) scores. **Results**: A total of 32 enzymatically debrided hands of 24 patients were included with a mean age of 42.4 ± 16.8 years and a mean follow-up of 31 months. Postoperatively, 19 of these could be managed conservatively using skin substitutes such as "Suprathel", 13 had to undergo subsequent autografting. The mean DASH score for the entire study population was eight with a mean value of four in the conservatively managed group and fourteen in the autografted group. The mean Patient, Observer POSAS, and VSS values were nineteen, thirteen, and two. A total of 30 cases showed an effortless complete fist closure, and, also in 30 cases, patients attested to be satisfied with the esthetic appearance of the hand on being asked. **Conclusions**: The descriptive analysis of these results in our study population suggests that the enzymatic debridement of deep burns of the hand, especially combined with subsequent conservative management with skin substitutes, was associated with low long-term hand disability scores at a follow-up of two years.

Keywords: enzymatic debridement; Nexobrid®; hand burns; hand function

1. Introduction

Over the past decade, bromelain-based enzymatic debridement has established itself as an effective and even superior alternative to conventional excisional debridement, preventing the necessity of escharotomy, reducing the number of burns requiring autografting, as well as reducing healing time from the first debridement [1–7]. In many clinics, it is steadily replacing conventional debridement as the standard of care in the treatment of deep dermal burns because of its selective ability to preserve (partially) viable dermal tissue and enhance the chances of spontaneous healing [4,8,9].

Hand burns are very common, being implicated in 30 to 90% of burn patients [2,10–12], and are an especially challenging field within burn treatment because of the hand's complex anatomy. Especially in this field, enzymatic debridement has been of great significance. Preserving viable dermal tissue in the hand, a complex anatomical instrument prone to developing contractures due to its many joints can be beneficial for maintaining normal hand function.

With an increasing number of burn victims surviving their injuries, the preservation of hand function becomes even more crucial for their quality of life [13]. Conventional excisional debridement in the form of tangential excision or hydrosurgery is very traumatic and inadvertently removes healthy dermal tissue with its capacity for spontaneous healing. The often-used aphorism "If epidermis is life, dermis is quality of life" is particularly pertinent in this field of burn surgery, for having one normally or nearly normally functioning hand can make the difference between being self-sufficient and being dependent on others in our daily activities.

The early and continuous intensive mobilization of the hand after deep burn injuries is essential for long-term hand function [10,12,14,15]. Enzymatic debridement seems to not only preserve viable dermal tissue optimizing the patient's own regeneration potential, but also spares the patient the postoperative hand immobilization. Studies evaluating long-term hand functionality after enzymatic debridement are scarce. These find similar or superior long-term functional results after enzymatic debridement in comparison to conventional debridement in adults [2,4,7]. In our study, we aimed to evaluate the long-term hand functionality in our adult patient population after the enzymatic debridement of deep dermal burns.

2. Materials and Methods

This study has been approved by our hospital's Institutional Review Board. A retrospective analysis was conducted on patients having undergone enzymatic debridement of the hands between 2015 and 2022 in our inpatient clinic (with 26 beds) or the intensive care unit for severe burns (with 6 beds) in "Nuremberg Hospital". "Klinikum Nuremberg" is a 2200-bed tertiary hospital.

2.1. Patient Inclusion

All cases of deep hand burns in which enzymatic debridement with Nexobrid® was applied were searched and identified in the clinics database using specific International Classification of Disease (ICD) codes. Our study population and this study only included patients over the age of 16. Patients with burns under the age of 16 are treated by pediatric surgeons in our clinic. We aimed to exclude individuals with rheumatoid diseases impacting the hands, as well as those with other hand traumas or a history of hand surgery that affected their hand function, as these conditions would introduce a potential bias. However, none had to be excluded for these reasons. A total of 38 patients had been selected and 24 of them were included in the study. For the remaining 14 patients, the distance from their home to our clinic was too far, they were unable to fit the visit into their schedule during the weeks when we were available to perform physical examinations, or the retrospective chart review showed too many significant missing variables (see the flowchart in Figure 1).

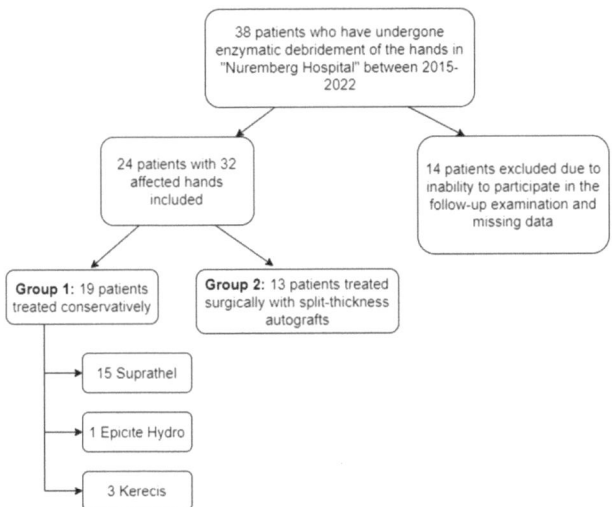

Figure 1. Flowchart of patients.

2.2. Standard Procedures in Regards to Enzymatic Debridement

On admission, the included patients with deep hand burns received wet wound dressings consisting of bandages rinsed in polyhexanide solution. These wet dressings were continued for at least 24 h as part of the presoaking regime. In our clinic, burns are diagnosed and designated using capillary refill testing as well as Laser Doppler Imaging (LDI).

Enzymatic debridement with Nexobrid® in our clinic follows European consensus guidelines [16,17]. Depending on the initial wound evaluation post-debridement (24–48 h), the following treatment paths were determined: superficial burns were treated conservatively through "Suprathel" application, while deep partial-thickness and mixed burns were treated conservatively with skin substitutes "Epicite Hydro" or "Kerecis". Full-thickness burns required split-thickness autologous skin grafting. Mixed-depth burns were also managed conservatively to promote spontaneous epithelialization (see flowchart in Figure 1). If healing was inadequate after 2 weeks, autografting was considered. Early mobilization was encouraged for the conservatively treated cases (starting on the first postoperative day), while the autografted hands were immobilized for 4–5 days postoperatively.

2.3. Data Collection and Final Routine Follow-Up Examination

A retrospective data analysis was performed including reviewing the patient files and photo and video documentation. In the period between March 2022 and August 2022, the included patients were invited to participate in a routine follow-up examination. During the routine follow-up examination, the patients were asked to fill out the Disabilities of the Arm, Shoulder, and Hand (DASH) [18,19], Patient and Observer Scar Assessment Scale (POSAS) [20,21], and Vancouver Scar Scale (VSS) [22] scores. Additionally, patients were interviewed regarding current symptoms, persisting disabilities during daily life, their professional situation, their medical history, and whether they were satisfied with the esthetic appearance of their affected hands or not. This examination included a detailed physical assessment of various aspects of hand function. The condition of the scars and any potential contractures were carefully evaluated. Sensitivity was assessed using the two-point discrimination test, a method that determines the ability to discern two close points on the skin. To evaluate thumb mobility, the opposition score as defined by Kapandji [23] was employed, which provides a standardized measure of thumb function. The range of motion (ROM) of both the metacarpophalangeal (MCP) and interphalangeal (IP) joints of the affected fingers was measured using a goniometer. Additionally, hand strength was assessed using specific tools. Pinch strength between the thumb and index finger was measured with the Jamar pinch gauge, which is designed to evaluate the force exerted in a person's pinch grip. Overall, handgrip strength was measured using the Jamar dynamometer, an instrument for assessing the maximum isometric strength of the hand and forearm muscles. Most importantly, patients were instructed to demonstrate full fist closure and full hand extension, both of which were documented photographically. The physical examinations were conducted by a fifth-year medical student under the direct supervision of the first author, following extensive practice of the procedures.

2.4. Statistical Analysis

The relatively low number of patients in the conservatively and surgically treated groups after enzymatic debridement caused a proper statistical analysis to be impossible. Therefore, only a descriptive analysis was performed.

3. Results

A total of 24 patients were included in this study, with 32 enzymatically debrided burned hands and with a mean follow-up of 31 months. The mean age of these patients was 42 years (ranging from 16 to 71), with twenty-one male and three female patients (Table 1). In eight patients, both hands were involved, and in nineteen patients, the dominant hand was involved. The mean total burned body surface area (TBSA) was 15%, ranging from 10 to 70%. A total of six hands had mixed burns with superficial partial-thickness being predominant; eighteen showed deep partial-thickness burns; and eight showed full-thickness burns. In the case of a mixed burn pattern, the predominant burn depth was documented. In 22 hand burns in our study, both the palm and the dorsum of the hand were involved.

Table 1. Patient characteristics presented with mean values and standard deviations. (Chronic obstructive pulmonary disease (COPD)).

	Total Study Population (n = 32)	Conservatively Treated Group 1 (n = 19)	Surgically Treated Group 2 (n = 13)
Age (years)	42.4 ± 16.8	43	41
Follow-up (months)	31.4 ± 17.1	32	31
Male sex	26	17	9
Total burned body surface area (%)	15.1 ± 15.3	10	23
Burn depth			
Superficial partial-thickness	6	6	0
Deep partial-thickness	18	12	6
Full-thickness	8	1	7
Palm of the hand involved	26	14	12
Dorsum of the hand involved	28	17	11
Renal insufficiency	4	3	1
Heart disease	0	0	0
Immunosuppression	0	0	0
COPD	3	3	0
Depression	1	1	0
Nicotine dependency	6	6	0

After enzymatic debridement, 19 hands were treated conservatively (group 1) and 13 hands surgically (group 2). Both groups did not show relevant differences in mean age or follow-up time and consisted of predominantly men. The mean TBSA was greater in group 2 with 23% vs. 10% in group 1. Also, group 2 included seven out of the total eight full-thickness burns. The palm of the hand seemed to be more frequently affected in group 2 (12/13 vs. 14/19).

Some observations in the Results Section warrant further clarification. Despite the study's primary focus on deep dermal burns, Table 1 indicates the inclusion of six superficial partial-thickness burns. This discrepancy arises from the classification of many mixed-depth burn cases by their predominant depth. Specifically, these six cases consisted of a mix of 60% superficial partial-thickness and 40% deep partial-thickness and/or full-thickness burns. None of these six mixed-depth burn cases had to be treated surgically.

3.1. Conservative vs. Surgical Treatment Following Enzymatic Debridement

A total of nineteen hand burns were treated conservatively, fifteen of which with "Suprathel", three of which with "Kerecis", and one with "Epicite Hydro" (Table 2). The 13 hand burns in group 2 were all treated surgically following enzymatic debridement through excisional debridement and split-thickness autografting. In twelve cases, the indication for ensuing surgical treatment was set directly at the post-enzymatic wound bed evaluation, and, in one case, after the failed conservative treatment.

Table 2. Specifics pertaining to the enzymatic debridement and the ensuing conservative or surgical treatments.

	Total Study Population ($n = 32$)	Conservatively Treated Group 1 ($n = 19$)	Surgically Treated Group 2 ($n = 13$)
Wound bed:			
Uniform pink/red	12	10	2
Uniform white + punctuate bleeding	18	7	11
Step-off/Depression	6	0	6
Exposed fatty tissue	4	0	4
Exposed thrombosed veins	6	1	5
Second applicatiion of Nexobrid®	0	0	0
Post-enzymatic application of			
Suprathel	15	15	0
Epicite Hydro	1	1	0
Kerecis	3	3	0
Split-thickness autograft	13	0	13

In 10 out of 12 cases where a pink or red wound bed evaluation (superficial partial-thickness burns) was observed, a conservative treatment also ensued. The two remaining cases, despite initially presenting with a uniform pink wound bed upon evaluation, exhibited delayed healing in the following 2 weeks and consequently required subsequent surgical treatment. Also, in all but one case where signs of full-thickness burns were identified (such as step-offs/depressions, exposed fatty tissue, and thrombosed veins), surgical treatment with split-thickness autografting ensued. A white wound bed with pin-point punctate bleeding (deep partial-thickness burns), occurring in eighteen cases, resulted in conservative treatment in seven of the cases and surgical treatment in eleven cases.

3.2. Questionnaire Scores

The mean DASH score was found to be eight for the entire study population (range 0–27), with a mean score of four in the conservatively treated group and a mean score of fourteen in the surgically treated group (Table 3, Figure 2). A total of nine patients (28%)

had a DASH score ≥ 15, eight of which were treated surgically and one conservatively. The DASH score seemed not to be age-dependent.

Table 3. Questionnaire scores and functional outcomes. Disabilities of the Arm, Shoulder, and Hand (DASH), Patient and Observer Scar Assessment Scale (POSAS), Vancouver Scar Scale (VSS).

	Total Study Population (n = 32)	Conservatively Treated Group 1 (n = 19)	Surgically Treated Group 2 (n = 13)
DASH (0–100)	8.4 ± 8.1	4	14
POSAS Patient (6–60)	18.5 ± 9.1	14	24
POSAS Observer (6–60)	12.9 ± 6.5	10	17
VSS (0–13)	2.4 ± 1.7	2	4
Complete fist closure			
possible	30	19	11
not possible	2	0	2
Kapandji Score (0–10)	10	10	9
Handgrip strength (kg)	35.8 ± 16.2	41	28
Pinch grip strength (kg)	7.1 ± 3.1	8	6

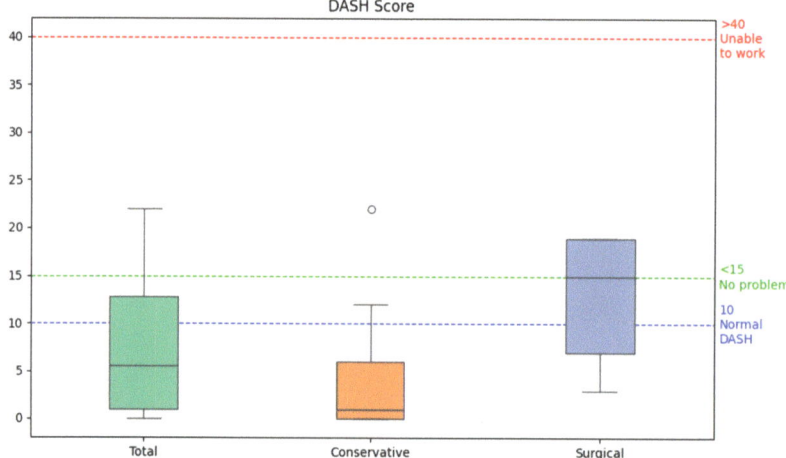

Figure 2. Boxplots for the Disabilities of the Arm, Shoulder, and Hand (DASH) score distribution of the conservatively and surgically treated groups following enzymatic debridement. The dot in the middle of the figure is an outlier value. The normal DASH score has been reported to be around 10 in a general population study [24]. The following cut-off values for the DASH score have been described: <15 corresponds with "no problem", 16–40 with "problem, but working", >40 with "unable to work" [25].

The mean patient POSAS score was 19 for the entire study population, with a mean value of 14 in the conservatively treated group and 24 in the surgically treated group. The mean values for the observer POSAS score were 13 for the entire study population, 10 in group 1, and 17 in group 2 (Table 3, Figure 3). The mean VSS score was two in the entire group, with a mean value of two in the conservatively treated patients and four in the surgically treated patients. A total of two patients attested not to be pleased with the esthetic appearance of their burned hand. Both of them were treated surgically following enzymatic debridement.

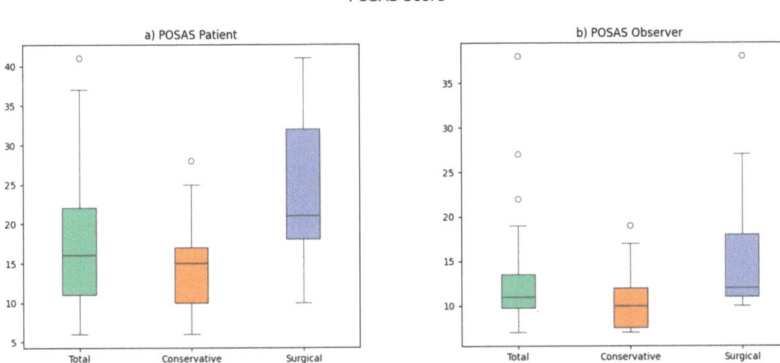

Figure 3. Boxplots for the Patient (**a**) and Observer (**b**) Scar Assessment Scale (POSAS) of the conservatively and surgically treated groups following enzymatic debridement. The dots represent outlier values.

3.3. Functional Results

In four cases, pain was reported involving the burned hand area (one case in group 1 and three cases in group 2). Cold intolerance was reported in fourteen cases, eight of which were in the surgically treated group. In 31 cases, a two-point discrimination between 4 and 6 mm was found. Scar contractures were seen in a total of nine burned hands, seven of which were in the surgically treated group. These included mostly interdigital contractures.

Nonetheless, in 30 of the 32 cases, the patient could demonstrate complete fist closure. Most hands showed an overall full range of motion, with nearly full extension and the abduction of the fingers. A maximum Kapandji score of ten was found in twenty-five hands and a score of nine was found in six hands. In one surgically treated hand, a Kapandji score of four was found. The mean handgrip strength was found to be 36 kg for the entire group, with 41 kg in group 1 and 28 kg in group 2 (Figure 4). The mean pinch grip strength was also lower in group 2 with 6 kg compared to 8 kg in group 1.

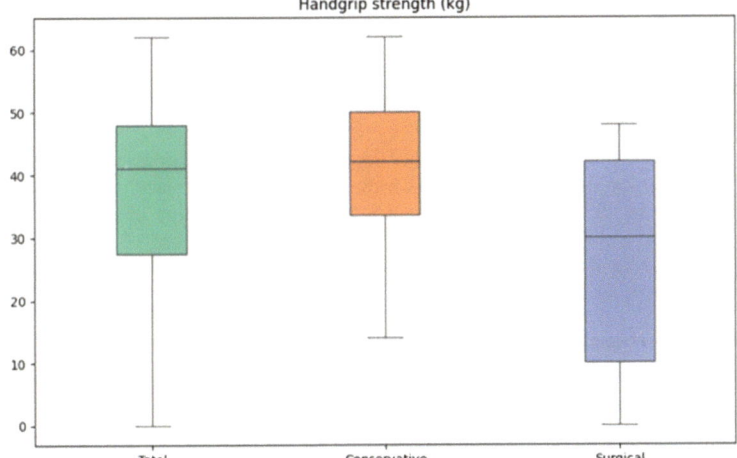

Figure 4. Boxplots for the handgrip strength of the conservatively and surgically treated groups following enzymatic debridement.

4. Discussion

In this study, we aimed to evaluate the long-term hand function after the enzymatic debridement of deep dermal burns through descriptively analyzing the following outcome measures and comparing them to the existing literature.

4.1. DASH

For the DASH questionnaire, we found a mean score of eight, (four in group 1, fourteen in group 2). Our mean DASH score of eight is beneath the score of ten, which was found in a general study population [24], and beneath the cut-off value of 15, which is considered unproblematic in the DASH score interpretation [25]. In a prospective study of 16 enzymatically debrided upper extremities, Cordts et al. found a mean DASH score of 23 at a 3-month follow-up [11]. This is relatively high in comparison to many other similar studies, which have a longer follow-up time, such as Fischer et al., who found a mean DASH of 13.9 in a prospective study of 20 enzymatically debrided upper extremities at a 12-month follow-up [3]. This role of the follow-up time is confirmed by Cherubino et al., finding a mean DASH of 21 at a 6-month follow-up and a mean DASH of 11 at a 15-month follow-up in 18 enzymatically debrided upper extremities [26]. Furthermore, Corrales-Benitez et al. prospectively found a mean DASH value of 0.2 in 90 enzymatically debrided hands [27]. Heitzmann et al. reported a mean DASH score of seven in thirty-one enzymatically debrided hands. Both of these were found at a mean follow-up of 12 months, which is very similar to our own results [4]. Despite the many inhomogeneities of these studies, they do seem to support the favorable DASH values found in our study, especially after a follow-up time of 12 months or longer.

4.2. POSAS and VSS

With a mean patient POSAS value of 19 and an observer POSAS value of 13, one could conclude that, in our study, the observers were generally more satisfied with the long-term scars than the patients were. However, the POSAS values suggest that both patient (POSAS of 14 in group 1 vs. 24 in group 2) and observer (POSAS of 10 in group 1 vs. 17 in group 2) seemed to be more satisfied with the scar quality after conservative post-enzymatic treatment than after surgical post-enzymatic treatment (Table 3). In the study by Cherubino et al., mean patient and observer POSAS values of 16 and 14 were reported [26]. Heitzmann et al. conducted a comparative study between 31 enzymatically and 15 surgically debrided hands, reporting patient and observer POSAS values of 21 and 17, respectively in the enzymatically debrided group, and of 33 and 26 in the surgically debrided group [4]. These patient and observer POSAS values suggest poorer scar quality after surgical debridement than after enzymatic debridement of hand burns and seem to correspond with our own results.

The mean VSS value of two (of thirteen) found in this study suggests an overall favorable subjective scar quality, with a worse score in the surgically treated group 2. The minimal difference in VSS scores between groups 1 and 2 (two vs. four), however, is not very interpretable. The aforementioned study by Cordts et al. finds a mean VSS score of six in enzymatically debrided hands [11], corresponding with a worse scar quality than in our study, however at a much shorter follow-up.

4.3. Fist Closure and Handgrip Strength

Only two of the thirty-two examined hands were unable to demonstrate a full fist closure at a mean follow-up of 31 months, suggesting a relatively good long-term hand function. Both of these hands were treated surgically post-enzymatically, arguing in favor of conservative post-enzymatic treatment. A general population study by Wang et al. in the USA reports a mean grip strength of 40 kg in the dominant hand of men [28]. Considering the fact that our study concerned injured hands of mostly men with 80% of the study population, a mean grip strength of 36 kg (41 kg in group 1 vs. 28 kg in group 2) seems acceptable. As of yet, the literature does not provide many studies reporting on the handgrip strength after enzymatic debridement.

In line with our findings, most of these previous studies [3,5,6,11,26,27,29], especially the ones comparing enzymatic debridement to the standard of care [1,2,4,7], find long-term functional and esthetic results which are equal or superior to conventional excisional debridement.

4.4. Conservative vs. Surgical Treatment Following Enzymatic Debridement

In this study, we were not able to compare enzymatically debrided hands to conventionally debrided hands; however, we were able to descriptively compare our subgroups consisting of the conservatively and surgically treated hand burns post-enzymatically. Most of the functional outcome measures in this study (Table 3) were worse in the surgically treated group following enzymatic debridement. In particular, the differences in DASH and POSAS scores, fist closure, and handgrip strength were noteworthy. The relatively high number of deep partial-thickness burns in the conservatively treated group suggests that, on initial presentation, seemingly deep burns can be managed conservatively, confirming the reduction in autografting after enzymatic debridement reported in previous studies [1,2,7].

However, to our knowledge, we seem to be the first to compare conservative and surgical treatment modalities following enzymatic debridement. We consistently found worse esthetic and functional results in the surgically treated group than in the conservatively treated group post-enzymatically. This corresponds with the trend seen in the comparison between primarily surgically debrided hand burns vs. primarily enzymatically debrided hand burns. This is illustrated, for instance, by the parallel between the better POSAS values in the conservatively treated group (14 and 10 in group 1 vs. 24 and 17 in group 2) in our study and the better POSAS values in the enzymatically debrided group (21 and 17 in the enzymatic group vs. 33 and 26 in the surgical group) in the study by Heitzmann et al. [4]. Therefore, a logical hypothesis seems to be that, when hand burns do require surgical treatment either indicated directly at presentation, after post-enzymatic wound bed evaluation, or after failed conservative treatment, the pretreatment through enzymatic debridement seems to become less important for long-term hand function for the surgical trauma of excisional debridement and the contracture potential of autografts remain the same. Therefore, the functional results of surgically treated hand burns post-enzymatically might be comparable to the functional results after the conventional surgical treatment of hand burns. Of course, this hypothesis warrants further research in a comparative study with conventionally surgically treated deep dermal hand burns.

4.5. Limitations

An important limitation of this study is its retrospective nature and the subsequent difficulties in obtaining homogenous data. This study has a relatively extended follow-up period of 31 months and focuses exclusively on enzymatically debrided hands.

However, for a statistical analysis, the sample size of both groups is too small to yield reliable statistical testing. Our conclusions are based on a descriptive analysis only, and should therefore be interpreted with caution. These trends need to be validated through future research involving larger sample sizes that would allow for meaningful statistical analysis. The absence of a control group consisting of primarily surgically debrided hand burns also poses a potential limitation, as mentioned above. Additionally, the greater mean TBSA and the number of full-thickness burns in group 2 pose a potential bias.

5. Conclusions

With a relatively low sample size, the enzymatic debridement of deep dermal hand burns in this study showed a promising trend in long-term functional results, especially if it is followed by conservative wound treatment using skin substitutes. With complete fist closure achieved in nearly all patients and mean DASH scores indicating low disability levels, we argue that enzymatic debridement is a viable treatment method for hand burns, where the preservation of dermal tissue can be crucial for the maintenance and restoration of hand function after deep dermal burns.

Author Contributions: Conceptualization, A.T.M., T.P., D.E. and P.I.H.; methodology, A.T.M., A.E.-H. and M.B. (Moritz Billner); software, A.E.-H., M.B. (Maresa Berns) and K.J.B.; validation, A.T.M., M.B. (Maresa Berns) and T.P.; formal analysis, A.T.M. and M.B. (Moritz Billner); investigation, A.T.M. and M.B. (Moritz Billner); resources, D.E. and K.J.B.; data curation, A.T.M. and A.E.-H.; writing—original draft preparation, A.T.M.; writing—review and editing, A.T.M., A.E.-H., M.B. (Moritz Billner), M.B. (Maresa Berns), T.P., K.J.B., P.I.H. and D.E.; visualization, A.T.M. and A.E.-H.; supervision, P.I.H. and D.E.; project administration, A.T.M. and M.B. (Maresa Berns). All authors have read and agreed to the published version of the manuscript.

Funding: This research received no external funding.

Institutional Review Board Statement: The study was conducted according to the guidelines of the Declaration of Helsinki, and approved by the Institutional Review Board of Nuremberg Hospital ("Klinikum Nürnberg") (protocol code: IRB-2022-004, approved on 4 March 2022).

Informed Consent Statement: Informed consent was obtained from all subjects involved in the study concerning a routine follow-up examination and the possible publication of the results.

Data Availability Statement: All the data analyzed during this study are available from the corresponding author on reasonable request.

Acknowledgments: We would like to acknowledge the administrative support provided by Lisa Angerer during the follow-up examinations in the out-patient clinic.

Conflicts of Interest: The authors declare no conflict of interest.

References

1. Rosenberg, L.; Krieger, Y.; Bogdanov-Berezovski, A.; Silberstein, E.; Shoham, Y.; Singer, A.J. A novel rapid and selective enzymatic debridement agent for burn wound management: A multi-center RCT. *Burns* **2014**, *40*, 466–474. [CrossRef]
2. Krieger, Y.; Rubin, G.; Schulz, A.; Rosenberg, N.; Levi, A.; Singer, A.J.; Rosenberg, L.; Shoham, Y. Bromelain-based enzymatic debridement and minimal invasive modality (mim) care of deeply burned hands. *Ann. Burns Fire Disasters* **2017**, *30*, 198–204.
3. Fischer, S.; Haug, V.; Diehm, Y.; Rhodius, P.; Cordts, T.; Schmidt, V.J.; Kotsougiani, D.; Horter, J.; Kneser, U.; Hirche, C. Feasibility and safety of enzymatic debridement for the prevention of operative escharotomy in circumferential deep burns of the distal upper extremity. *Surgery* **2019**, *165*, 1100–1105. [CrossRef]
4. Heitzmann, W.; Schulz, A.; Fuchs, P.C.; Schiefer, J.L. Assessing the Effect of Enzymatic Debridement on the Scar Quality in Partial-Thickness Burns to Deep Dermal Burns of the Hand: A Long-Term Evaluation. *Medicina* **2024**, *60*, 481. [CrossRef]
5. Dadras, M.; Wagner, J.M.; Wallner, C.; Sogorski, A.; Sacher, M.; Harati, K.; Lehnhardt, M.; Behr, B. Enzymatic debridement of hands with deep burns: A single center experience in the treatment of 52 hands. *J. Plast. Surg. Hand Surg.* **2020**, *54*, 220–224. [CrossRef] [PubMed]
6. Schulz, A.; Perbix, W.; Shoham, Y.; Daali, S.; Charalampaki, C.; Fuchs, P.C.; Schiefer, J. Our initial learning curve in the enzymatic debridement of severely burned hands—Management and pit falls of initial treatments and our development of a post debridement wound treatment algorithm. *Burns* **2017**, *43*, 326–336. [CrossRef] [PubMed]
7. Schulz, A.; Shoham, Y.; Rosenberg, L.; Rothermund, I.; Perbix, W.; Fuchs, P.C.; Lipensky, A.; Schiefer, J.L. Enzymatic versus traditional surgical debridement of severely burned hands: A comparison of selectivity, efficacy, healing time, and three-month scar quality. *J. Burn Care Res.* **2017**, *38*, e745–e755. [CrossRef]
8. Shoham, Y.; Gasteratos, K.; Singer, A.J.; Krieger, Y.; Silberstein, E.; Goverman, J. Bromelain-based enzymatic burn debridement: A systematic review of clinical studies on patient safety, efficacy and long-term outcomes. *Int. Wound J.* **2023**, *20*, 4364–4383. [CrossRef] [PubMed]
9. Rosenberg, L.; Krieger, Y.; Silberstein, E.; Arnon, O.; Sinelnikov, I.A.; Bogdanov-Berezovsky, A.; Singer, A.J. Selectivity of a bromelain based enzymatic debridement agent: A porcine study. *Burns* **2012**, *38*, 1035–1040. [CrossRef]
10. Pan, B.S.; Vu, A.T.; Yakuboff, K.P. Management of the acutely burned hand. *J. Hand Surg. Am.* **2015**, *40*, 1477–1484. [CrossRef]
11. Cordts, T.; Horter, J.; Vogelpohl, J.; Kremer, T.; Kneser, U.; Hernekamp, J.F. Enzymatic debridement for the treatment of severely burned upper extremities—Early single center experiences. *BMC Dermatol.* **2016**, *16*, 8. [CrossRef] [PubMed]
12. Lehnhardt, M.; Hartmann, B.; Reichert, B. (Eds.) *Verbrennungschirurgie*, 1st ed.; Springer: Berlin/Heidelberg, Germany, 2016.
13. Sheridan, R.L.; Hurley, J.; Smith, M.A.; Ryan, C.M.; Bondoc, C.C.; Quinby, W.C., Jr.; Tompkins, R.G.; Burke, J.F. The acutely burned hand: Management and outcome based on a ten-year experience with 1047 acute hand burns. *J. Trauma Acute Care Surg.* **1995**, *38*, 406–411. [CrossRef] [PubMed]

14. Gant, T.D. The early enzymatic debridement and grafting of deep dermal burns to the hand. *Plast. Reconstr. Surg.* **1980**, *66*, 185–190. [CrossRef] [PubMed]
15. Schneider, J.C.; Qu, H.D.; Lowry, J.; Walker, J.; Vitale, E.; Zona, M. Efficacy of inpatient burn rehabilitation: A prospective pilot study examining range of motion, hand function and balance. *Burns* **2012**, *38*, 164–171. [CrossRef]
16. Hirche, C.; Citterio, A.; Hoeksema, H.; Koller, J.; Lehner, M.; Martinez, J. Eschar removal by bromelain based enzymatic debridement (Nexobrid) in burns: AN European consensus. *Burns* **2017**, *43*, 1640–1653. [CrossRef] [PubMed]
17. Hirche, C.; Almeland, S.K.; Dheansa, B.; Fuchs, P.; Governa, M.; Hoeksema, H.; Korzeniowski, T.; Lumenta, D.B.; Marinescu, S.; Martinez-Mendez, J.R.; et al. Eschar removal by bromelain based enzymatic debridement (Nexobrid®) in burns: European consensus guidelines update. *Burns* **2020**, *46*, 782–796. [CrossRef] [PubMed]
18. Soohoo, N.F.; McDonald, A.P.; Seiler, J.G., 3rd; McGillivary, G.R. Evaluation of the construct validity of the DASH questionnaire by correlation to the SF-36. *J. Hand Surg. Am.* **2002**, *27*, 537–541. [CrossRef] [PubMed]
19. Copeland, A.; Gallo, L.; Weber, C.; Moltaji, S.; Gallo, M.; Murphy, J.; Axelrod, D.; Thoma, A. Reporting Outcomes and Outcome Measures in Thumb Carpometacarpal Joint Osteoarthritis: A Systematic Review. *J. Hand Surg.* **2021**, *46*, 65.e1–65.e11. [CrossRef] [PubMed]
20. Draaijers, L.J.; Tempelman, F.R.H.; Botman, Y.A.M.; Tuinebreijer, W.E.; Middelkoop, E.; Kreis, R.W.; van Zuijlen, P.P.M. The patient and observer scar assessment scale: A reliable and feasible tool for scar evaluation. *Plast. Reconstr. Surg.* **2004**, *113*, 1960–1965, Discussion 6–7. [CrossRef]
21. van de Kar, A.L.; Corion, L.U.; Smeulders, M.J.; Draaijers, L.J.; van der Horst, C.M.; van Zuijlen, P.P.M. Reliable and feasible evaluation of linear scars by the Patient and Observer Scar Assessment Scale. *Plast. Reconstr. Surg.* **2005**, *116*, 514–522. [CrossRef]
22. Sullivan, T.; Smith, J.; Kermode, J.; McIver, E.; Courtemanche, D.J. Rating the burn scar. *J. Burn Care Rehabil.* **1990**, *11*, 256–260. [CrossRef] [PubMed]
23. Kapandji, A. [Clinical test of apposition and counter-apposition of the thumb]. *Ann. Chir. Main. Organe Off. Soc. Chir. Main.* **1986**, *5*, 67–73. [CrossRef] [PubMed]
24. Hunsaker, F.G.; Cioffi, D.A.; Amadio, P.C.; Wright, J.G.; Caughlin, B. The American academy of orthopaedic surgeons' outcomes instruments: Normative values from the general population. *J. Bone Jt. Surg. Am.* **2002**, *84*, 208–215. [CrossRef] [PubMed]
25. Angst, F.; Schwyzer, H.K.; Aeschlimann, A.; Simmen, B.R.; Goldhahn, J. Measures of adult shoulder function: Disabilities of the Arm, Shoulder, and Hand Questionnaire (DASH) and its short version (QuickDASH), Shoulder Pain and Disability Index (SPADI), American Shoulder and Elbow Surgeons (ASES) Society standardized shoulder assessment form, Constant (Murley) Score (CS), Simple Shoulder Test (SST), Oxford Shoulder Score (OSS), Shoulder Disability Questionnaire (SDQ), and Western Ontario Shoulder Instability Index (WOSI). *Arthritis Care Res.* **2011**, *63* (Suppl. S11), S174–S188.
26. Cherubino, M.; Valdatta, L.; Baroni, T.; Pellegatta, I.; Tamborini, F.; Garutti, L.; Di Summa, P.; Adani, R. Selective Enzymatic Debridement for The Management of Acute Upper Limb Burns. *Ann. Burns Fire Disasters* **2021**, *34*, 328–333. [PubMed]
27. Corrales-Benítez, C.; González-Peinado, D.; González-Miranda, Á.; Martínez-Méndez, J.R. Evaluation of burned hand function after enzymatic debridement. *J. Plast. Reconstr. Aesthetic Surg.* **2022**, *75*, 1048–1056. [CrossRef]
28. Wang, Y.C.; Bohannon, R.W.; Li, X.; Sindhu, B.; Kapellusch, J. Hand-grip strength: Normative reference values and equations for individuals 18 to 85 years of age residing in the United States. *J. Orthop. Sports Phys. Ther.* **2018**, *48*, 685–693. [CrossRef]
29. Krieger, Y.; Bogdanov-Berezovsky, A.; Gurfinkel, R.; Silberstein, E.; Sagi, A.; Rosenberg, L. Efficacy of enzymatic debridement of deeply burned hands. *Burns* **2012**, *38*, 108–112. [CrossRef]

Disclaimer/Publisher's Note: The statements, opinions and data contained in all publications are solely those of the individual author(s) and contributor(s) and not of MDPI and/or the editor(s). MDPI and/or the editor(s) disclaim responsibility for any injury to people or property resulting from any ideas, methods, instructions or products referred to in the content.

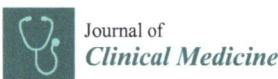

Case Report

Flap-Free Tendon Coverage Using Autologous Fat Grafts Enhanced with Platelet-Rich Plasma and Growth Factors at a Secondary Level Hospital: A Case Report

Guadalupe Santamaría Salvador [1], Esteban Acosta Muñoz [2], Juan Samaniego Rojas [1], Charles Hidalgo Quishpe [1], Juan S. Izquierdo-Condoy [2], Jorge Vasconez-Gonzalez [2] and Esteban Ortiz-Prado [2],*

[1] Plastic and Reconstructive Department, Hospital Vozandes, Quito 170521, Ecuador
[2] One Health Research Group, Faculty of Health Science, Universidad de Las Americas, Quito 170513, Ecuador
* Correspondence: e.ortizprado@gmail.com

Abstract: Background: Autologous fat grafting, enriched with platelet-rich plasma (PRP), has been established as an effective and affordable treatment for various types of wound healing. However, its efficacy in managing wounds with tendon exposure has not been thoroughly investigated. Methods: We report the case of a 40-year-old male who sustained a severe friction burn on his hand and forearm from a car accident, resulting in significant tissue loss and exposed extensor tendons. Results: Traditional wound treatment strategies were not implemented due to specific patient circumstances. After initial surgical management failed to prevent necrosis and maintain coverage of the exposed tendons, the patient underwent a novel treatment involving autologous fat grafting combined with PRP and growth factors. The procedure was repeated twice within a month to promote granular tissue formation over that area and facilitate subsequent coverage with an epidermoreticular graft. By day 21 post-initial graft, the exposed tendons were 98% covered with granular tissue. Complete wound coverage was achieved by day 60, and by day 130 the patient had regained 90% functionality of the affected limbs. Conclusions: This case illustrates the potential of autologous fat grafting combined with PRP and growth factors as a viable, flap-free alternative for covering tendon exposures. This approach not only enhances wound healing but also supports functional recovery, underscoring the need for further research into its broader applicative potentials.

Keywords: autologous fat graft; tendon exposure; platelet-rich plasma; wound healing; regenerative medicine

1. Introduction

Fat grafting, commonly referred to as "lipofilling," is a sophisticated surgical procedure that involves the transfer of autologous adipose tissue from one bodily region to another [1]. This technique, facilitated through minimally invasive liposuction, not only proves to be well-tolerated by patients but also stands as a safe and effective approach for various therapeutic and aesthetic applications [2]. Recent advancements have highlighted adipose tissue as a rich reservoir of adult stem cells—more concentrated than any other tissue type—which exhibit potential for cellular differentiation across various tissue types, including adipose, bone, muscle, cartilage, nervous, and vascular tissues [3]. The stromal vascular fraction (SVF) within adipose tissue is particularly valued for its reparative and regenerative capabilities [4,5].

With the rapid development of transportation and construction industries, skin and subcutaneous soft tissue defects have become increasingly common. Such injuries often result in the exposure of critical underlying structures such as tendons and bones, posing significant clinical challenges. The treatment of large and refractory wounds requires advanced soft tissue management techniques to avoid complications like infection, scar contracture, and potentially, disability [6–8]. These scenarios typically necessitate interventions that range from simple second-intention healing to more complex procedures like skin grafting with or without dermal substitutes, or local to distant flaps [6–9].

Conventional treatments often involve debridement followed by the transplantation of skin flaps [10]. However, this can result in significant donor site morbidity and may not be suitable due to the poor vascularity, reduced tissular partial pressure of oxygen (PtO2) at the defect sites, or reduced local growth factor activity [11,12]. Platelet-rich plasma (PRP), a regenerative biomaterial, has gained attention for its high concentrations of growth factors such as platelet-derived growth factor (PDGF), transforming growth factor-beta (TGF-β), and vascular endothelial growth factor (VEGF), which promote angiogenesis and tissue repair at the defect sites [13,14]. When combined with autologous fat grafting, PRP not only enhances the survival of the grafted tissue but also supports angiogenesis and cellular differentiation, making this combination a potent option for managing complex wounds [15,16].

This study explores the therapeutic potentials of autologous fat grafting combined with PRP in the treatment of a severe case involving tendon exposure following a traffic accident. The case underscores the challenges of healing poorly vascularized defects and the innovative application of combined regenerative therapies to facilitate functional recovery and aesthetic improvement.

2. Case Report

A 40-year-old male with no significant personal or family medical history was presented to the emergency department following a traffic accident that resulted in trauma to his left hand and forearm. The injuries occurred when his left upper limb was forcibly displaced and came into contact with the pavement.

Upon stabilization in the emergency department, the patient was evaluated for fractures, which were ruled out. The plastic surgery team conducted a thorough examination, revealing a significant friction burn on the left hand and forearm, with a tissue loss area measuring approximately 8 cm × 7 cm on the dorsum of the left hand. Additionally, there was a detachment of the extensor aponeurotic system involving the second to fifth tendons. A separate wound, 5 cm × 2.5 cm, was found on the ulnar border of the left forearm. An avulsion injury to the cortex of the distal epiphysis of the radius was also noted. No signs of compartment syndrome were present (Figure 1).

2.1. Initial Management and Surgical Intervention

Upon admission, the patient was promptly started on antibiotic therapy with a combination of Ampicillin and Sulbactam at a dosage of 3 g to prevent infection. Within six hours of the accident, the patient underwent surgery, where extensive debridement was performed to clean the wound. Tenorrhaphy of the second to fifth extensor tendons was completed using the Bunnell technique. The wound on the dorsum of the hand was primarily closed with the remaining perilesional skin. The hand was immobilized in a 90-degree hyperextension using an anterior splint, which was to remain in place for 15 days. The wound edges on the forearm were approximated and closed by secondary intention to prevent compartment syndrome.

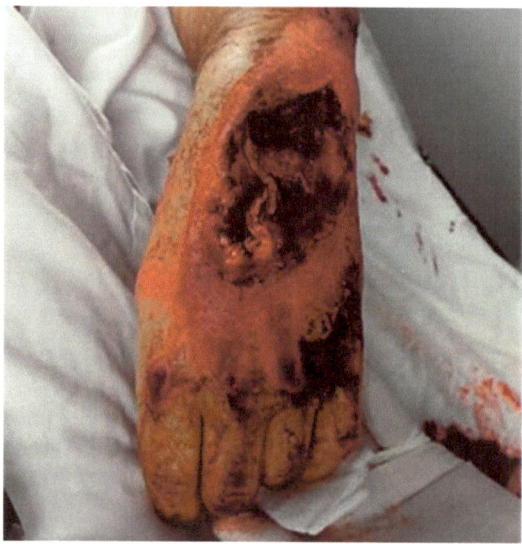

Figure 1. Initial clinical presentation of the left hand and forearm injuries. This image displays extensive trauma to the patient's left hand and forearm resulting from a traffic accident. Visible are the friction burn and the subsequent loss of skin measuring 8 cm × 7 cm on the dorsum of the hand. This figure also shows a detachment of the extensor aponeurotic system from the second to fifth tendons, along with a 5 cm × 2.5 cm wound located on the ulnar border of the forearm's middle third. Notable is the avulsion of the cortex of the distal epiphysis of the radius. The exposed tendons and surrounding muscle tissues are clearly delineated, highlighting the complex nature of the injuries sustained.

2.2. Postoperative Care

Fifteen minutes post-surgery, the splint was temporarily removed to check for any signs of circulatory or nerve compression before being reapplied. Four days post-surgery, irrigation was performed with 500 cc of 0.9% saline solution, and the hydrocolloid bandage (Duoderm) was changed. This process was repeated every four days. Wound cultures were performed every eight days until the first fat graft, all of which were negative for bacterial superinfection. Physical therapy began on the fifth day, following an early mobilization protocol to prevent damage to other structures due to the hyperextension position of the hand. The hyperextension splint was changed to a dynamic splint in the first week. Physical therapy included four phases: immobilization and early controlled mobilization (0–3 weeks), active-assisted mobilization (4–6 weeks), full active mobilization (7–12 weeks), and strengthening with a return to full function (13 weeks onwards).

2.3. Complication Management

On the twenty-ninth day following surgery, a 4 × 4 cm area of necrosis with tendon exposure was identified on the dorsum of the affected hand, involving the second to fourth extensor tendons, accompanied by perilesional granulation tissue (Figure 2). The patient declined further surgical interventions such as local or free microsurgical skin flap. Consequently, it was decided to treat the exposed tendons using an autologous fat graft augmented with PRP and growth factors, aiming to leverage their regenerative capabilities.

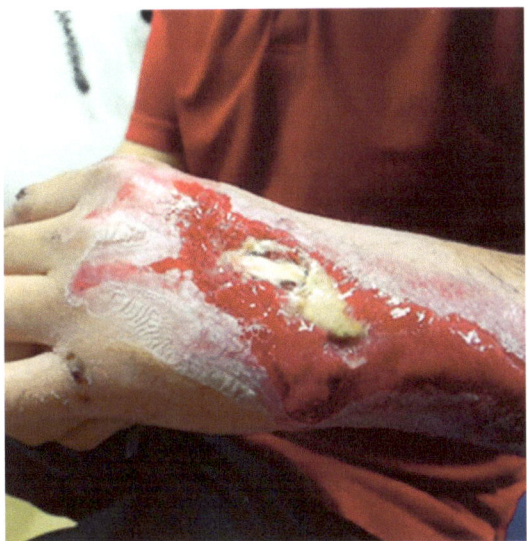

Figure 2. Initial postoperative necrosis with exposed tendons and granulation tissue.

2.4. Autologous Fat Grafting Technique and Platelet-Rich Plasma Preparation

The required instruments for the fat graft pooling technique included saline solution (0.9%), epinephrine (dilution 1:1,000,000), bicarbonate, 2% lidocaine, a 3 mm liposuction cannula for fat grafting, a 10 cc syringe (vacuum syringe), and Vaseline gauze.

Autologous fat was harvested from the abdominal panniculus, specifically the periumbilical area, during both the first and second sessions. The donor site was infiltrated using a tumescent technique with a solution of 0.9% saline, 1:1,000,000 epinephrine, 10 mEq of bicarbonate, and 10 cc of 2% lidocaine without epinephrine. A 3 mm liposuction cannula was then used to harvest approximately 10 cc of fat tissue per session. The harvested fat was processed via decantation in the same collection syringe for 3 min. The lower portion was then removed, isolating the fat. The isolated fat was then mixed with 5 cc of PRP activated with 1 cc of thrombin to release growth factors. The procedure described corresponded to the preparation of platelet-rich plasma (PRP), which was activated with thrombin at the time of use to promote the release of growth factors.

Blood Collection: Venipuncture was performed to collect between 15 and 20 cc of the patient's blood into 3.5 mL tubes containing sodium citrate as an anticoagulant (blue cap). The volume of blood collected may vary depending on the patient's hematocrit. In this case, the patient's hematocrit was 45.5%, which is within the typical range of 40–50% for a healthy young male.

Centrifugation: The tubes were centrifuged immediately after collection at high speeds (6000–8000 rpm) for 15 min at room temperature. Following centrifugation, the blood was fractionated and the plasma was extracted while avoiding leukocytes.

Platelet Count: While the hospital protocol does not include an individualized platelet count for the PRP, it is estimated, based on institutional experience, that the platelet concentration in PRP is approximately five times higher than in peripheral blood. In this case, the patient had a peripheral blood platelet count of 206,000 platelets per microliter.

PRP Activation: To activate the platelets in PRP and facilitate the release of growth factors such as platelet-derived growth factor (PDGF), transforming growth factor-beta (TGF-β), and vascular endothelial growth factor (VEGF), a secondary protocol, termed "Obtaining Autologous Thrombin," was followed.

This procedure was performed at the time of PRP use. Blood was collected from the patient into tubes without additives (red cap) with volumes ranging from 15 to 20 cc.

The tube was centrifuged at a low speed (4000 rpm) for 10 min at room temperature. Subsequently, a fibrin clot was formed, and thrombin was obtained from the residual serum. For activation, the protocol specifies using between 0.5 cc and 1 cc of thrombin. In this case, 1 cc of thrombin was utilized, and it is important to note that calcium chloride was not employed in this procedure.

The mixture of autologous fat and PRP was applied to Vaseline gauze, which was then placed over the exposed tendons on the dorsum of the hand, specifically covering the 4 × 4 cm area of necrosis with tendon exposure. This was further covered with saline-soaked gauze and then with a gauze bandage. Concurrently, partial-thickness epidermoreticular (ER) grafts were placed adjacent to the necrotic area over the granulating tissue to promote skin regeneration on the dorsum of the affected hand and over the wound located in the middle third of the left forearm along the ulnar border, which was initially managed by secondary intention to prevent compartment syndrome (Figure 3).

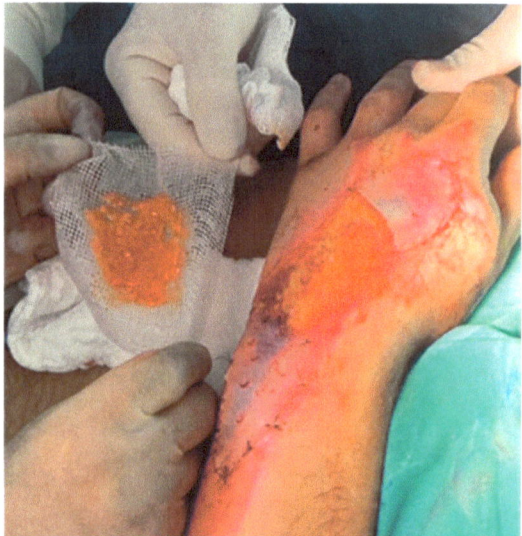

Figure 3. Application of autologous fat graft in the middle third (4 × 4 cm area of necrosis with tendon exposure on the dorsum of the affected hand, involving the second to fourth extensor tendons) and partial-thickness ER grafts in the lateral thirds (adjacent to the necrotic areas).

2.5. Follow-Up and Outcome

Three days after the initial fat graft application, 50% graft vitality was noted, prompting a second application of adipose tissue combined with PRP and growth factors, particularly targeting the necrotic areas. By the fourth day following this second intervention, graft vitality had improved to 90%. Hydrocolloid dressings were maintained until approximately 98% tissue degranulation was achieved, followed by a final ER grafting. Sixty days post-second grafting, complete wound coverage was observed.

At 130 days after the first surgical intervention, although specific range-of-motion measurements for each tendon were not performed, functional recovery was deemed satisfactory based on the patient's ability to perform daily activities without significant restrictions or pain. The patient denied experiencing weakness, pain, paresthesias, or sensory loss in the back of the forearm and hand, except in the area where the first and second autologous fat grafts were performed, which exhibited some sensory loss. No muscle atrophy was observed in the muscles innervated by the radial and posterior interosseous nerves. The patient was able to perform full functional flexion and extension movements in the second to fifth fingers (Supplementary Material S1). Elbow extension against resistance, wrist extension, and thumb extension against resistance were normal, with no sign of dropped wrist evident. Sensitivity was preserved in the back of the arm, forearm, and hand (first interdigital space), except in the aforementioned area. The patient's self-assessment indicated a 90% recovery of functionality (Figure 4). The DASH questionnaire in the disability scoring module yielded a score of 12, indicating low disability (Supplementary Material S2). Although the traumatologists recommended surgical correction for the avulsion injury to the cortex of the distal epiphysis of the radius, the patient declined, given that his hand functionality in daily activities was not affected, and the integrity of the achieved skin coverage was a priority.

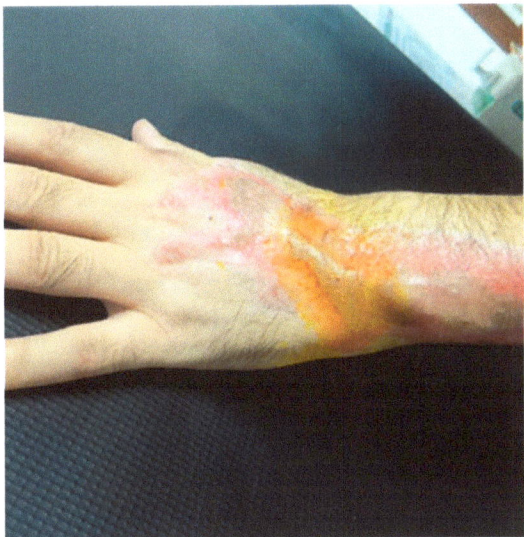

Figure 4. Final result of healing showing complete wound coverage accompanied by functional recovery.

3. Discussion

This report details the outcomes of using autologous fat grafting augmented with PRP and growth factors to manage a wound with exposed tendons resulting from a traffic accident, a scenario that poses considerable healing challenges. Traditional approaches, such as local or remote skin flaps, are often preferred for primary wound repair, especially in cases involving poorly vascularized defects like exposed bones or tendons [15]. However, due to the unique characteristics of the lesion and the patient's preference against conventional flap techniques, these methods were not suitable.

Instead, a novel approach involving autologous fat grafting combined with PRP and growth factors was employed, offering a promising alternative that facilitated significant functional recovery. The primary advantage of this technique lies in the rich presence of connective tissue cells within the stromal vascular fraction of adipose tissue, which includes a diverse cell population such as preadipocytes, endothelial cells, monocytes, macrophages, granulocytes, lymphocytes, and notably, adipose-derived stem cells (ADSCs). These cells are integral to promoting wound healing through mechanisms like enhanced cellular proliferation, differentiation, reduced inflammation, and improved vascularization [16–18].

The procedure's low invasiveness and ease of access further reduce the risks associated with more invasive sources like bone marrow [11,12]. Additionally, the role of PRP in accelerating the healing process of traumatic wounds and ulcers is well-established, with benefits stemming from the high concentration of platelet-derived growth factors enhancing tissue repair and angiogenesis [19,20]

Despite these advantages, the technique is not devoid of potential complications, which can include bleeding, infection, and, in rare cases, graft hypertrophy from excessive collagen deposition [21]. Extensive testing in both animal and human clinical studies has validated the efficacy of autologous fat grafting combined with PRP across various wound types and anatomical locations. Yet, the literature remains scant on its application in wounds with significant tendon exposure, as demonstrated in this case [22–24].

This gap is notable, although the technique has been explored for other applications such as filling depressed scars and covering bone exposures. For instance, Kao et al. reported that fat grafts, used alongside negative pressure therapy, facilitated mesenchymal healing in a murine model, creating enough granulation tissue for effective bone coverage suitable for subsequent skin grafting [25]. Similarly, Rangaswamy M. described successful outcomes in a series involving patients with bone exposure using the same intervention strategy [26].

These findings from animal models underscore the potential of autologous fat graft and PRP therapy in complex clinical scenarios involving exposed tissues that carry functional risks, such as bones and tendons. The absence of extensive clinical reports using this regenerative therapy as a tissue bridge in deep wounds highlights the innovative aspect of our approach and underscores the need for further research. This would not only validate the efficacy and safety of this technique but also refine its application protocols, maximizing therapeutic outcomes in clinical practice.

From a public health perspective, traditional wound care methods, such as prolonged use of colloid patches, hydrocolloids, alginate dressings, and platelet gels, often require extensive resource utilization over long treatment periods [27,28]. These conventional treatments can become economically burdensome due to the high costs of long-term care and frequent dressing changes required to manage chronic wounds. Furthermore, they may lead to delayed reintegration into the workforce due to prolonged recovery times.

In contrast, the use of autologous fat grafts combined with PRP offers a more efficient solution via potentially reducing the healing time and improving the functional recovery of patients. This not only minimizes direct medical costs through curtailing the need for repetitive and extensive wound management resources but also mitigates indirect costs associated with lost productivity and prolonged disability. Moreover, through preventing complications such as infection or chronic pain that often accompany traditional treatments, this approach could further reduce the likelihood of long-term healthcare expenditures.

Enhancing the regenerative capabilities of wound care through such innovative therapies could substantially alleviate the public health burden of treating complex injuries. It could enable quicker patient recovery and a faster return to work, which are critical components in improving quality of life and reducing the economic impact on both individuals and healthcare systems. Therefore, advancing this technique through rigorous research could have profound implications for public health policy and clinical practices worldwide.

4. Limitations

While this study offers valuable insights into the potential benefits of autologous fat grafting combined with platelet-rich plasma and growth factors, there are several inherent limitations due to its clinical case design. The surgical approach used—autologous fat grafting—was an alternative to the standard treatment (local or free microsurgical skin flap), chosen because the patient declined the standard treatment. Additionally, the current literature on the use of autologous fat grafting as an alternative to flaps for tendon exposure coverage in the upper extremity is limited, which restricts the scope of discussion in this report and underscores its significance. It is important to note that platelet counting was not performed on the platelet-rich plasma preparations in accordance with established protocols, though incorporating this step could enhance the accuracy of the procedure's replication and potentially improve the success rate of similar cases. Lastly, the plastic surgery team did not employ negative pressure therapy, given their limited experience with autologous fat grafting as an alternative to flaps for tendon coverage in the upper extremity.

Despite the possibility of achieving similar results in a shorter time via combining fat grafting with negative pressure, this report remains valuable as it highlights a successful outcome in a constrained setting.

5. Conclusions

Autologous fat tissue graft combined with PRP and growth factors has proven to be a highly effective alternative to traditional flap procedures for covering exposed tendons. This method not only facilitates skin regeneration but also positively influences the behavior of dermal and epidermal cells through the bioactive compounds in its "secretome". The technique's relative ease of access, cost-effectiveness, nonimmunogenic nature, and potential to enhance aesthetic outcomes make it an attractive option in clinical scenarios involving tissue exposure. Its application could revolutionize the approach to wound healing in plastic and reconstructive surgery, providing a simpler, quicker, and potentially less costly alternative to more invasive methods.

Supplementary Materials: The following supporting information can be downloaded at: https://www.mdpi.com/article/10.3390/jcm13185640/s1, Supplementary Material S1: Video S1: Full Functional Recovery: Demonstrating Complete Flexion and Extension in Fingers 2–5. Supplementary Material S2: Patient responses to DASH questionnaire.

Author Contributions: G.S.S. managed the patient throughout the treatment process and was primarily responsible for the patient's care. E.A.M., J.S.R. and C.H.Q. assisted in patient management, collected photographs, and contributed to patient care. J.S.I.-C. prepared the initial draft of the manuscript, J.V.-G., J.S.I.-C. and E.O.-P. reviewed and revised the manuscript critically for important intellectual content and wrote the final version of the manuscript. All authors have read and agreed to the published version of the manuscript.

Funding: This research received no external funding.

Institutional Review Board Statement: Not applicable.

Informed Consent Statement: Informed consent was obtained from all the subjects involved in this study.

Data Availability Statement: Due to the nature of this case report, the data supporting the findings cannot be shared publicly in order to protect patient confidentiality. However, further details may be made available by the corresponding author upon reasonable request.

Conflicts of Interest: The authors declare that the research was conducted in the absence of any commercial or financial relationship that could be construed as a potential conflict of interest.

References

1. Costanzo, D.; Romeo, A.; Marena, F. Autologous Fat Grafting in Plastic and Reconstructive Surgery: An Historical Perspective. *Eplasty* **2022**, *22*, e4. [PubMed]
2. Doornaert, M.; Colle, J.; De Maere, E.; Declercq, H.; Blondeel, P. Autologous fat grafting: Latest insights. *Ann. Med. Surg.* **2018**, *37*, 47–53. [CrossRef] [PubMed]
3. Smith, O.J.; Jell, G.; Mosahebi, A. The use of fat grafting and platelet-rich plasma for wound healing: A review of the current evidence. *Int. Wound J.* **2018**, *16*, 275–285. [CrossRef] [PubMed]
4. Shauly, O.; Gould, D.J.; Ghavami, A. Fat Grafting: Basic Science, Techniques, and Patient Management. *Plast. Reconstr. Surg. Glob. Open* **2022**, *10*, e3987. [CrossRef] [PubMed]
5. Colonna, M.R.; Scarcella, M.C.; do Stagno d'Alcontres, F.; Delia, G.; Lupo, F. Should fat graft be recommended in tendon scar treatment? Considerations on three cases (two feet and a severe burned hand). *Eur. Rev. Med. Pharmacol. Sci.* **2014**, *18*, 753–759.
6. Zuk, P.A.; Zhu, M.; Ashjian, P.; De Ugarte, D.A.; Huang, J.I.; Mizuno, H.; Alfonso, Z.C.; Fraser, J.K.; Benhaim, P.; Hedrick, M.H. Human adipose tissue is a source of multipotent stem cells. *Mol. Biol. Cell* **2002**, *13*, 4279–4295. [CrossRef]
7. Coleman, S.R. Structural fat grafting: More than a permanent filler. *Plast. Reconstr. Surg.* **2006**, *118*, 108S–120S. [CrossRef]
8. Deptula, P.; Block, T.; Tanabe, K.; Kulber, D. Autologous Fat Grafting in the Upper Extremity: Defining New Indications. *Plast. Reconstr. Surg. Glob. Open* **2022**, *10*, e4469. [CrossRef]
9. Ring, A.; Beutel, H.; Kirchhoff, P.; Bushart, S.U.; Dellmann, N.-C.; Farzaliyev, F. Rekonstruktion posttraumatischer sprunggelenknaher Weichteildefekte durch freie Faszienlappen aus dem anterolateralen Oberschenkel. *Unfallchirurgie* **2023**, *126*, 136–144. [CrossRef]

10. Namgoong, S.; Jung, S.-Y.; Han, S.-K.; Kim, A.-R.; Dhong, E.-S. Clinical experience with surgical debridement and simultaneous meshed skin grafts in treating biofilm-associated infection: An exploratory retrospective pilot study. *J. Plast. Surg. Hand Surg.* 2020, *54*, 47–54. [CrossRef]
11. Ortiz-Prado, E.; Dunn, J.F.; Vasconez, J.; Castillo, D.; Viscor, G. Partial pressure of oxygen in the human body: A general review. *Am. J. Blood Res.* 2019, *9*, 1. [PubMed]
12. Hu, K.; Olsen, B.R. The roles of vascular endothelial growth factor in bone repair and regeneration. *Bone* 2016, *91*, 30–38. [CrossRef] [PubMed]
13. Mazzucco, L.; Borzini, P.; Gope, R. Platelet-derived factors involved in tissue repair—From signal to function. *Transfus. Med. Rev.* 2010, *24*, 218–234. [CrossRef] [PubMed]
14. Demidova-Rice, T.N.; Durham, J.T.; Herman, I.M. Wound Healing Angiogenesis: Innovations and Challenges in Acute and Chronic Wound Healing. *Adv. Wound Care* 2012, *1*, 17–22. [CrossRef] [PubMed]
15. Morris, D. Overview of Flaps for Soft Tissue Reconstruction—UpToDate. Available online: https://www.uptodate.com/contents/overview-of-flaps-for-soft-tissue-reconstruction (accessed on 28 March 2024).
16. Ueberreiter, K. Autologous Fat Tissue Transfer, 1st ed.Springer: Cham, Switzerland, 2019.
17. Modarressi, A. Platlet Rich Plasma (PRP) Improves Fat Grafting Outcomes. *World J. Plast. Surg.* 2013, *2*, 6–13.
18. Toyserkani, N.M.; Quaade, M.L.; Sørensen, J.A. Cell-Assisted Lipotransfer: A Systematic Review of Its Efficacy. *Aesthetic Plast. Surg.* 2016, *40*, 309–318. [CrossRef]
19. Carruthers, J.; Humphrey, S. Injectable Soft Tissue Fillers: Permanent Agents—UpToDate. Available online: https://www.uptodate.com/contents/injectable-soft-tissue-fillers-permanent-agents (accessed on 28 March 2024).
20. Segreto, F.; Marangi, G.F.; Nobile, C.; Alessandri-Bonetti, M.; Gregorj, C.; Cerbone, V.; Gratteri, M.; Caldaria, E.; Tirindelli, M.C.; Persichetti, P. Use of platelet-rich plasma and modified nanofat grafting in infected ulcers: Technical refinements to improve regenerative and antimicrobial potential. *Arch. Plast. Surg.* 2020, *47*, 217–222. [CrossRef]
21. Chicharro-Alcántara, D.; Rubio-Zaragoza, M.; Damiá-Giménez, E.; Carrillo-Poveda, J.M.; Cuervo-Serrato, B.; Peláez-Gorrea, P.; Sopena-Juncosa, J.J. Platelet Rich Plasma: New Insights for Cutaneous Wound Healing Management. *J. Funct. Biomater.* 2018, *9*, 10. [CrossRef]
22. Benjamin, M.A.; Schwarzman, G.; Eivazi, M.; Zachary, L. Autologous staged fat tissue transfer in post-traumatic lower extremity reconstruction. *J. Surg. Case Rep.* 2015, *2015*, rjv141. [CrossRef]
23. Picard, F.; Hersant, B.; La Padula, S.; Meningaud, J.-P. Platelet-rich plasma-enriched autologous fat graft in regenerative and aesthetic facial surgery: Technical note. *J. Stomatol. Oral Maxillofac. Surg.* 2017, *118*, 228–231. [CrossRef]
24. El Khoury, J.; Awaida, C.; Nasr, M.; Hokayem, N. Platelet-rich plasma and fat grafting for the treatment of inferior alveolar nerve neuropathy: The first case report. *Oral Maxillofac. Surg. Cases* 2017, *3*, 107–111. [CrossRef]
25. Shalaby, H.; El-Shawadfy, S. Correction of Depressed Scars with PRP Enriched Fat Graft. *Egypt. J. Plast. Reconstr. Surg.* 2018, *42*, 245–250. [CrossRef]
26. Kao, H.-K.; Hsu, H.-H.; Chuang, W.-Y.; Chang, K.-P.; Chen, B.; Guo, L. Experimental study of fat grafting under negative pressure for wounds with exposed bone. *Br. J. Surg.* 2015, *102*, 998–1005. [CrossRef] [PubMed]
27. Kus, K.J.B.; Ruiz, E.S. Wound Dressings—A Practical Review. *Curr. Dermatol. Rep.* 2020, *9*, 298–308. [CrossRef]
28. Sood, A.; Granick, M.S.; Tomaselli, N.L. Wound Dressings and Comparative Effectiveness Data. *Adv. Wound Care* 2014, *3*, 511–529. [CrossRef]

Disclaimer/Publisher's Note: The statements, opinions and data contained in all publications are solely those of the individual author(s) and contributor(s) and not of MDPI and/or the editor(s). MDPI and/or the editor(s) disclaim responsibility for any injury to people or property resulting from any ideas, methods, instructions or products referred to in the content.

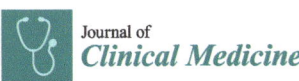

Article

Lipedema: Complications in High-Volume Liposuction Are Linked to Preoperative Anemia

Tonatiuh Flores [1,2,*], Barbara Kremsner [1], Jana Schön [1], Julia Riedl [3], Hugo Sabitzer [1,2], Christina Glisic [1,2], Kristina Pfoser [1,2], Jakob Nedomansky [1,2], Konstantin D. Bergmeister [1,2,4] and Klaus F. Schrögendorfer [1,2]

- [1] Karl Landsteiner University of Health Sciences, Dr. Karl-Dorrek-Straße 30, 3500 Krems, Austria; barbara.kremsner@oegk.at (B.K.); jana.schoen@gmx.net (J.S.); hugo.sabitzer@stpoelten.lknoe.at (H.S.); christina.glisisc@stpoelten.lknoe.at (C.G.); kristina.pfoser@stpoelten.lknoe.at (K.P.); jakob.nedomansky@stpoelten.lknoe.at (J.N.); konstantin.bergmeister@stpoelten.lknoe.at (K.D.B.); klaus.schroegendorfer@stpoelten.lknoe.at (K.F.S.)
- [2] Clinical Department of Plastic, Aesthetic and Reconstructive Surgery, University Clinic of St. Poelten, 3100 St. Poelten, Austria
- [3] Department of Medicine I, Division of Hematology and Hemostaseology, Medical University of Vienna, 1090 Vienna, Austria; julia.riedl@meduniwien.ac.at
- [4] Clinical Laboratory for Bionic Extremity Reconstruction, University Clinic for Plastic, Reconstructive and Aesthetic Surgery, Medical University of Vienna, 1090 Vienna, Austria
- * Correspondence: tonatiuh.flores@stpoelten.lknoe.at; Tel.: +43-2742-9004-23624

Abstract: Background: Lipedema is a subcutaneous adipose tissue disorder mainly affecting women. Its progressive nature often requires high-volume liposuction for efficient pain reduction. However, aspiration volumes of more than 5 L within a single session may lead to a variety of complications. Thus, we examined the effect of high-volume liposuctions on lipedema patients and the incidence of associated complications. **Methods:** We analyzed perioperative differences in lipedema patients undergoing low- or high-volume liposuctions. Statistical analyses were performed, investigating postoperative complications and the correlation of patients' BMI, total amount of aspiration, duration of surgery, hospital stay and hemoglobin alterations. Complications were investigated according to the Clavien–Dindo Classification. Patients were divided in two groups based on the volume aspirated at liposuction (low-volume vs. high-volume liposuction). **Results:** Overall, 121 sessions were investigated. Mean total volume of aspiration was 8227.851 mL ± 3643.891. Mean preoperative hemoglobin levels were 13.646 g/dL ± 1.075 g/dL. Preoperatively, 7.44% of patients were anemic (Hb < 12 g/dL). Mean postoperative hemoglobin was 10.563 g/dL ± 1.230 g/dL. Postoperatively, 90.10% of patients showed Hb levels below 12 g/dL. Hemoglobin loss differed significantly between the two groups ($p = 0.001$). Significant correlations between pre- ($p = 0.015$) and postoperative ($p < 0.001$) hemoglobin levels and pre- ($p < 0.001$) and postoperative ($p < 0.001$) anemia with Class II complications were also seen. The total volume of aspiration did not correlate with complication rates ($p = 0.176$). **Conclusions:** Complication rates in high-volume liposuctions are hemoglobin-dependent rather than volume-associated. Preoperative anemia was the most influential for the occurrence of postoperative complications. To safely conduct high-volume liposuctions in lipedema patients, adequate patient selection and preoperative patient preparation are imperative.

Keywords: lipedema; hemoglobin loss; patient safety; high-volume liposuction

1. Introduction

Lipedema is a subcutaneous tissue disorder affecting adipocytes, predominantly encountered in women [1–3]. First described by Allen and Hines in 1940, it presents as a disproportionate accumulation of adipose tissue in upper and lower limbs. Pathological inflammation of subcutaneous tissue entails fibrotic alterations and pain, resulting in symmetrical swelling of the limbs, omitting the hands and feet [4–7]. Lipedema is often confounded in the case of obesity due to the increased body mass index (BMI) attributed to the presence of swollen extremities [2,8,9]. Additionally, it is resistant to modern diets and lifestyle changes [2,8–12].

Because of disease progression, many patients already suffer from advanced stages of lipedema, thus requiring high-volume liposuction (liposuction above 5 L of total aspirate per session) [7,13,14]. Thereby, lipedema reduction can be sufficiently addressed while conducting only few surgeries, even when upper and lower extremities are affected [15,16]. Yet, high-volume liposuctions may lead to various side-effects or complications [16,17]. Increased blood loss, Vitamin D depletion, or prolonged pain are encountered most frequently [7,16]. Thus, in this paper, we analyze high-volume liposuctions in lipedema patients on account of perioperative patient safety. We further aimed to disclose the feasibility of high-volume liposuction in lipedema patients. This research intends to support physicians safely performing high-volume liposuction in maximum-care facilities.

2. Materials and Methods

2.1. Study Design and Patient Analysis

In our study, we analyzed liposuctions of the lower extremities in lipedema patients between 1 January 2018 and 30 April 2021 at the Department of Plastic, Aesthetic and Reconstructive Surgery at the University Clinic of St. Poelten. The study was carried out as a retrospective, single-center study. Data were collected pseudonymously and adhered to Austrian data protection legislation. A standardized mean follow-up of one year was carried out at our department. Approval was granted by the ethics committee from the local institutional review board at the Karl Landsteiner University of Health Sciences Krems (reference number: ECS 1041/2021). The analyzed study data include the patient's age, the duration of surgery, the patient's BMI, the length of hospital stay, pre- and postoperative hemoglobin values (hb), dosage and duration of antithrombotic prophylaxis, infiltration volume and volume of aspiration during the liposuction. Further, we analyzed postoperatively encountered complications in concordance with the Clavien–Dindo Classification system. A 5-scale grading system was used to rank complications based on the therapy needed. It assists in stratifying the severity of complications, as a reliable and uniform tool. While Class III and IV entail surgical intervention, Class I and II only require pharmacological support (e.g., blood transfusions in Class II). Class V describes the patient's death. Anemia was disclosed as values below 12 g/dL according to the WHO classification [18]. Adiposity was defined as a BMI > 30 kg/m^2 according to the WHO classification [19].

2.2. Operative Procedure

In our institution, liposuction is performed under general anesthesia with the tumescence technique. Preoperatively, patients are examined and the areas requiring treatment are marked while standing for accurate identification. Antibiotic prophylaxis is administrated at least 30 min before the primary surgical incision and continued for one week postoperatively. Patients either receive 2.2 g of amoxicillin/clavulanic acid (Curam®, Sandoz GmbH, 6250 Kundl, Austria) or 600 mg of clindamycin (Dalacin®, Fareva Amboise Zone Industrielle, Routes des Industries 29, 37530 Pocé-sur-Cisse, France) in case of a penicillin allergy. For liposuction, we install a modified Klein's solution with 1000 mL Ringer's lactate (Ringer lactate®, Fresenius Kabi, Rue du Rempart 6, 27400 Louviers, France) containing one milliliter of 1:1000 epinephrin (Suprarenin® Sanofi-Aventis GmbH, 65926 Frankfurt am Main, Germany). The solution is infiltrated through small stab incisions placed at strategically selected locations by using a number eleven blade. These incisions are placed in areas easy to conceal postoperatively, e.g., by the patients clothing. After fifteen minutes of indwelling time for the tumescent solution to set, vibration-assisted liposuction (VAL) is performed using 3 and/or 4 mm multiport cannulas (multiport rapid extraction cannula, Moeller Medical® GmbH, Wasserkuppenstraße 29–31, 36043 Fulda, Germany) paired with a Moeller's liposuction device (Moeller Vibrasat Pro, Moeller medical® GmbH, Wasserkuppenstraße 29–31, 36043 Fulda, Germany).

After liposuction, the incisions are rinsed with Octenisept® (Schülke & Mayr GmbH, Robert-Koch-Straße 2, 22851, Norderstedt, Germany) and Skinsept® (Ecolab Germany GmbH, Ecolab-Allee 1, 40789 Monheim am Rhein, Germany) followed by plaster coating. Stab incisions are not sutured at our department, to allow for the tumescence solution to drain. Compression garments are applied while the patient is still in the operating room. Compression must be worn continuously, day and night, for the following three months. Patients receive antibiotic shielding for an additional seven days postoperatively and antithrombotic prophylaxis using low molecular heparin for 10 to 30 days postoperatively. Patients additionally receive 500–1500 mL saline solution by default at the ward.

2.3. Statistical Analyses

All collected patient data in the selected timeframe were pseudonymized. Data protection management was performed adhering to Austrian legislation. The collection and processing of the necessary patient information was carried out using Microsoft Excel (version 2010, Microsoft, Redmond, WA, USA, Version 4.2.0 for Windows (22 April 2022). Statistical analyses were conducted with IBM SPSS Statistics for Windows Version (Version 29, IBM, Armonk, NY, USA). Nominal data were described with absolute frequencies and percentages, while metric data were summarized using means and standard deviations. Further analyses investigating the impact of complications on postoperative patient recovery, *t*-tests for independent samples, and Spearman-Rho correlation analyses were performed. Results were considered significant in the case of $p < 0.05$.

3. Results

3.1. Demographics

Within our study we analyzed 184 liposuction sessions in 107 patients suffering from lipedema. Here, 38 liposuctions were excluded, as they were performed on the upper extremities, so as to not distort the dataset and to accurately compare our groups. Additionally, 25 sessions were excluded due to a lack of data (postoperative hemoglobin levels acquired after 48 h of surgery). Finally, 121 liposuctions in 90 patients met our criteria and were included in this study. Our dataset included exclusively women. Patients were further divided upon receiving low-volume liposuction (total volume aspirated ≤ 5 L) or high-volume liposuctions (total volume aspirated > 5 L). In total, 25 (20.66%) sessions of low-volume liposuction were performed, and 96 (79.34%) of high-volume liposuction.

Patients mean age was 39.969 years ± 12.244 years (Table 1). Mean overall BMI was 32.013 kg/m^2 ± 7.135 kg/m^2. Overall, 81 (66.94%) patients showed a BMI > 30 kg/m^2. Hospital stay was on average 4.27 days ± 1.08 days. The mean duration of surgery was 112.363 min ± 27.877 min. The total amount of infiltration was 7363.636 mL ± 2423.633 mL. The mean total volume of aspiration was 8227.851 mL ± 3643.891 mL. The mean preoperative hemoglobin level was 13.646 g/dL ± 1.075 g/dL. Postoperative hemoglobin had a mean of mean 10.563 g/dL ± 1.230 g/dL. The mean hemoglobin loss was 3.052 g/dL ± 1.191 g/dL. The duration of antithrombotic prophylaxis using low-molecular heparin had a mean of 18.50 days ± 11.51 days. Antithrombotic dosages had a mean of 43.801 mL ± 8.684 mL.

In total, 20 (16.52%) sessions were associated with postoperative complications adhering to the Clavien–Dindo Classification. Hereby, 2 (1.65%) were seen in patients experiencing low-volume liposuction (≤5 L aspirate) and 18 (14.88%) were seen in women experiencing high-volume liposuction (>5 L aspirate).

Table 1. Demography of patients included in this study.

Patient Characteristics		Lipoaspirate < 5 L	Lipoaspirate > 5 L	Total
Number		25 (20.66%)	96 (79.34%)	121
Age (years)	Mean Min–Max STD	42.52 23–66 ±12.965	39.30 19–72 ±12.031	39.969 19–72 ±12.244
BMI (kg/m^2)	Mean Min–Max STD	28.304 19.7–37.9 ±5.523	32.978 21–58.40 ±7.213	32.013 19.70–58.40 ±7.135
Duration of Surgery (min)	Mean Min–Max STD	94.920 45–189 ±31.303	116.906 70–207 ±25.162	112.363 45–207 ±27.877
Hospital Stay (days)	Mean Min–Max STD	4.000 3–8 ±1.000	4.343 2–11 ±1.103	4.272 2.0–11 ±1.087
Volume of Infiltration (mL)	Mean Min–Max STD	4952.000 1100–6000 ±1366.296	7991.666 2000–14,000 ±2240.332	7363.636 2000.00–14,000.00 ±2423.633
Volume of Aspiration (mL)	Mean Min–Max STD	3844.800 1570–5000 ±897.339	9369.270 5050–18,800 ±3193.211	8227.851 1570.00–18,800.00 ±3643.891
Hemoglobin, preoperative (g/dL)	Mean Min–Max STD	13.296 11.5–16.0 ±1.060	13.700 10.5–16.5 ±1.069	13.646 10.5–16.5 ±1.075
Hemoglobin, postoperative (g/dL)	Mean Min–Max STD	10.924 7.4–13.4 ±1.109	10.469 7.1–14.1 ±1.247	10.563 7.1–14.1 ±1.230
Hemoglobin Loss (g/dL)	Mean Min–Max STD	2.372 0.5–5.7 ±1.264	3.230 1.1–6.4 ±1.111	3.052 0.5–6.4 ±1.191
Anemia, preoperative	N	4 (16%)	5 (5.21%)	9
Anemia, postoperative	N	22 (88%)	87 (90.63%)	109
Antithrombosis prophylaxis dosage (mL)	Mean Min–Max STD	40.000 40–40 ±0.000	44.791 40–80 ±9.512	43.801 40–80 ±8.684
Antithrombosis prophylaxis duration (days)	Mean Min–Max STD	11.200 5–14 5.972	20.406 6–56 ±11.858	18.504 5–56 ±11.509

3.1.1. Low-Volume Liposuction

In total, 25 liposuctions were performed with an aspiration volume of less than or equal to 5 L. The mean age was 42.52 years ± 12.965 years. The mean duration of surgery in this group was 94.920 min ± 31.303 min. Total infiltration had a mean of 4952.00 mL ± 1366.296 mL. The mean volume of aspiration was 3844.800 ± 897.339 mL. Hospital stay had a mean of 4.00 days ± 1.000 day in this group. BMI had a mean of 28.304 kg/m^2 ± 5.523 kg/m^2. In this group, 15 patients (60%) had BMI > 25 kg/m^2. Preoperative hemoglobin was 13.296 g/dL ± 1.060 g/dL. Here, four (16%) women showed preoperative anemia. Postoperative hemoglobin was 10.924 g/dL ± 1.109 g/dL, with 22 (88%) patients experiencing postoperative anemia. Antithrombotic prophylaxis was given on mean for 11.20 days ± 5.97 days. The mean low-molecular heparin dosage was 40.000 mL.

Postoperative complications in low-volume patients were solely Class I. The main complications were slight dizziness and emesis, which required the use of antiemetics, presumably as a consequence of anesthesia. All complications ceased within 12 h and were not present at time of discharge.

3.1.2. High-Volume Liposuction

In this group, 96 women experienced liposuction above 5 L in total. The mean patient age was 39.30 years ± 12.031 years. The duration of surgery was 116.906 min ± 25.162 min on average. The total infiltration had a mean of 7991.666 mL ± 2240.332 mL. The mean volume of aspiration was 9369.270 ± 3193.211 mL. Hospital stay length had a mean of 4.35 days ± 1.10 days in this group. The mean BMI was 32.978 kg/m^2 ± 7.213 kg/m^2. Women experiencing high-volume liposuction showed a BMI > 25 kg/m^2 in 83 (86.46%) cases. Preoperative hemoglobin was 13.700 g/dL ± 1.069 g/dL. Here, five (5,21%) patients had preoperative anemia. Postoperative hemoglobin was 10.469 g/dL ± 1.247 g/dL, with 87 (90.63%) women experiencing postoperative anemia. Antithrombotic prophylaxis was obtained based on the mean of 20.41 days ± 11.86 days. The mean low-molecular heparin dosage was 44.791 mL ± 9.512 mL.

High-volume liposuction patients experienced 14 (11.57%) Class I complications, involving requiring only antiemetics or electrolytes. All Class I complications ceased after 12 h and where not present at time of discharge. The remaining four (3.30%) patients experienced Class II complications. Here, all patients received one blood transfusion postoperatively due to hemoglobin drop below 7.6 g/dL and hemodynamic manifestation. Two of the patients receiving blood transfusion had a history of varicose.

3.2. Statistical Analyses

3.2.1. Volume-Associated Statistical Analyses

Although our groups were unevenly distributed, statistical analyses were feasible. Statistical results proved to be significant, as sufficient data were present to entail reliable statistical power. Thus, a power analysis was not necessary. Due to the division of our patients into low-volume and high-volume liposuction, statistical analyses involving t-tests of independent samples showed obvious significances when analyzing liposuction volumes. The total volume of infiltration and aspiration differed significantly ($p < 0.01$) (Figure 1).

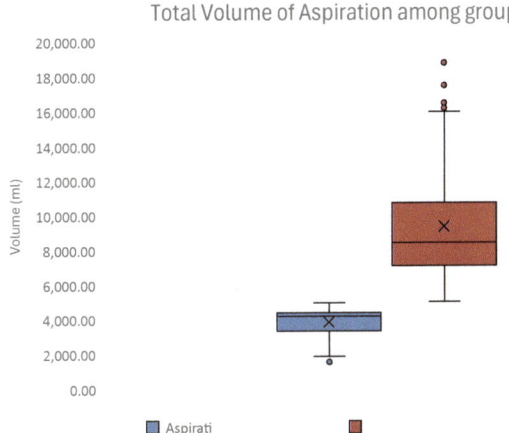

Figure 1. Boxplot of the total volume of aspiration between groups. As women were grouped into low-volume (≤5 L total aspiration) and high-volume (>5 L total aspiration) liposuction, minimum, maximum and mean values differed significantly ($p < 0.01$). Although statistically significant, these results show no clinical relevance. Women experiencing low-volume liposuction are displayed in blue; women experiencing high-volume liposuction are displayed in red. Outliers can be seen as dots.

3.2.2. Surgery-Associated Statistical Analyses

Comparing the duration of surgery between our groups, a statistical significance could be observed. Women experiencing high-volume liposuction showed significantly higher surgery time than women experiencing low-volume liposuction ($p < 0.001$) (Table 2). Although this finding was expected, the means of the duration of surgery between our groups are not as far apart as anticipated (Figure 2).

Table 2. Levene's Test analyzing duration of surgery between groups. Our analyses showed a significant difference in the duration of surgery between low- and high-volume liposuction ($p < 0.001$).

	Levene's Test of Equality of Variances						
	F	Sig.	T	df	One-sided p	Two-sided p	Mean difference
Duration of Surgery	0.818	0.368	−3.693	119	<0.001	<0.001	−21.986

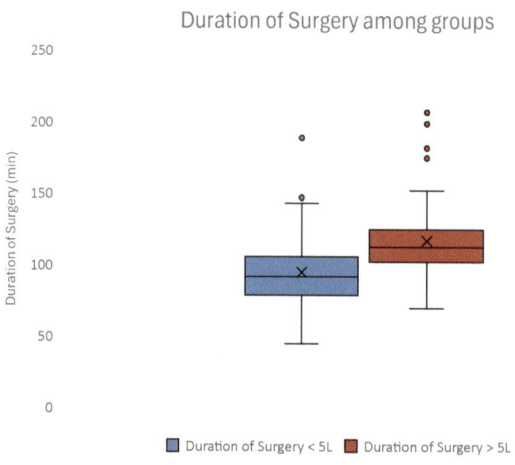

Figure 2. Boxplot of duration of surgery among groups. Women experiencing high-volume liposuction had significantly higher duration of surgery ($p < 0.001$). Women experiencing low-volume liposuction are displayed in blue; women experiencing high-volume liposuction are displayed in red. Outliers can be seen as dots.

No statistical significance between in-hospital durations ($p = 0.160$) was observed. Yet, when performing Spearman Rho analyses to correlate duration of surgery to hospital stay, we observed a statistical significance ($p = 0.019$) demonstrating that a longer duration of surgery significantly extends hospital stay (Table 3, Figure 3).

Table 3. Spearman Rho Rank analysis showing that duration of surgery has a significant impact on hospital stay ($p = 0.019$).

	Spearman Rho Correlation Analysis				
				Duration of Surgery	Hospital Stay
Spearman Rho	Duration of Surgery	Corr. Coefficient		1.000	0.213
		Sig. (2-tailed)			0.019
		N		121	121
	Hospital Stay	Corr. Coefficient		0.213	1.000
		Sig. (2-tailed)		0.019	
		N		121	121

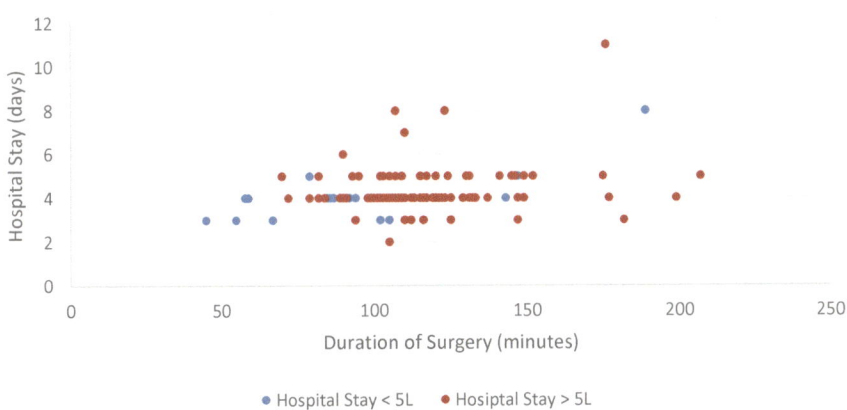

Figure 3. Scatter plot correlating duration of surgery to hospital stay, showing an extension in hospital stay with longer surgery times. A significant correlation can be observed ($p = 0.019$). Women experiencing low-volume liposuction are displayed in blue; women experiencing high-volume liposuction are displayed in red.

Further, higher total aspiration volumes directly extend hospital stay ($p < 0.001$) (Table 4).

Table 4. Spearman Rho Rank analysis showing that total volume of aspiration has a significant impact on hospital stay ($p < 0.001$).

		Spearman Rho Correlation Analysis		
			Volume total Aspiration	Hospital Stay
Spearman Rho	Volume total Aspiration	Corr. Coefficient	1.000	0.335
		Sig. (2-tailed)		<0.001
		N	121	121
	Hospital Stay	Corr. Coefficient	0.335	1.000
		Sig. (2-tailed)	<0.001	
		N	121	121

3.2.3. Patient-Associated Statistical Analyses

Conducting *t*-test analyses, no significant difference regarding BMI ($p = 0.03$) and age ($p = 0.243$) between our groups was seen. Our analyses of preoperative hemoglobin levels also showed no significance ($p = 0.094$). Postoperative hemoglobin values did not differ significantly either ($p = 0.100$) (Figure 4). There was also no significant difference in preoperative ($p = 0.178$) or postoperative anemia ($p = 0.699$) between low- and high-volume liposuction patients.

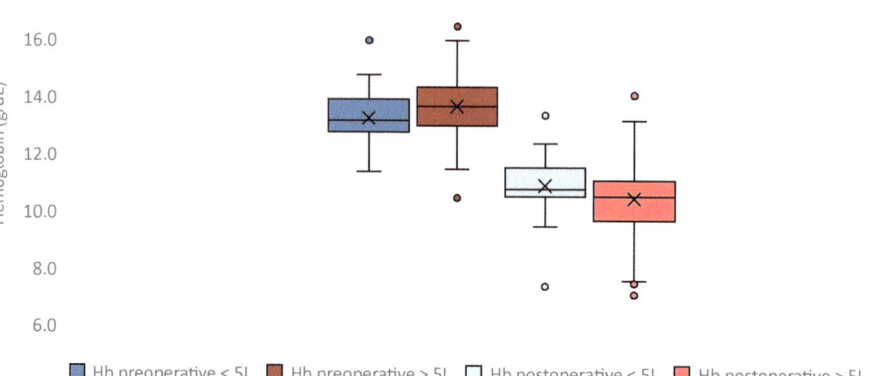

Figure 4. Boxplot of pre- and postoperative hemoglobin values. *t*-test analyses showed no statistical significance within either group. Women experiencing low-volume liposuction are displayed in blue; women experiencing high-volume liposuction are displayed in red. Outliers can be seen as dots.

Yet, hemoglobin loss between low- and high-volume liposuction patients did differ significantly ($p = 0.001$), demonstrating that high-volume liposuction sessions entail higher blood-loss than low-volume liposuction sessions (Table 5, Figure 5).

Table 5. Levene's Test showing a statistical significance regarding hemoglobin loss between both groups ($p < 0.001$).

	Levene's Test of Equality of Variances						
	F	Sig.	T	df	One-sided p	Two-sided p	Mean difference
Hemoglobin Loss	0.166	0.685	−3.341	119	<0.001	0.001	−0.858

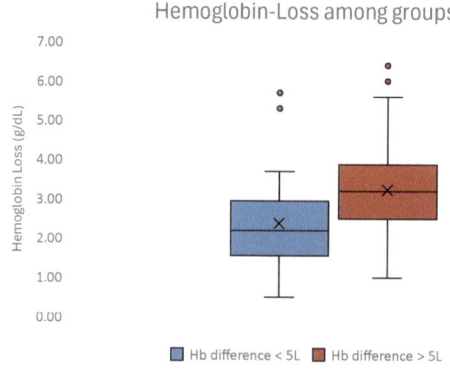

Figure 5. Boxplot of hemoglobin loss between both groups. Statistical analyses showed a significant difference regarding hemoglobin loss ($p = 0.001$). Women experiencing low-volume liposuction are displayed in blue; women experiencing high-volume liposuction are displayed in red. Outliers can be seen as dots.

Comparing both groups, no significance in postoperative complication rate adhering to the Clavien–Dindo Classification could be seen ($p = 0.122$). Performing analyses correlating hemoglobin loss to total aspiration volume, we observed a significant correlation ($p = 0.012$) (Table 6, Figure 6).

Table 6. Spearman Rho Rank analysis showing that total volume of aspiration has a significant impact on hemoglobin loss ($p = 0.012$).

		Spearman Rho Correlation Analysis		
			Volume total Aspiration	Hemoglobin Loss
Spearman Rho	Volume total Aspiration	Corr. Coefficient	1.000	0.227
		Sig. (2-tailed)		0.012
		N	121	121
	Hemoglobin Loss	Corr. Coefficient	0.227	1.000
		Sig. (2-tailed)	0.012	
		N	121	121

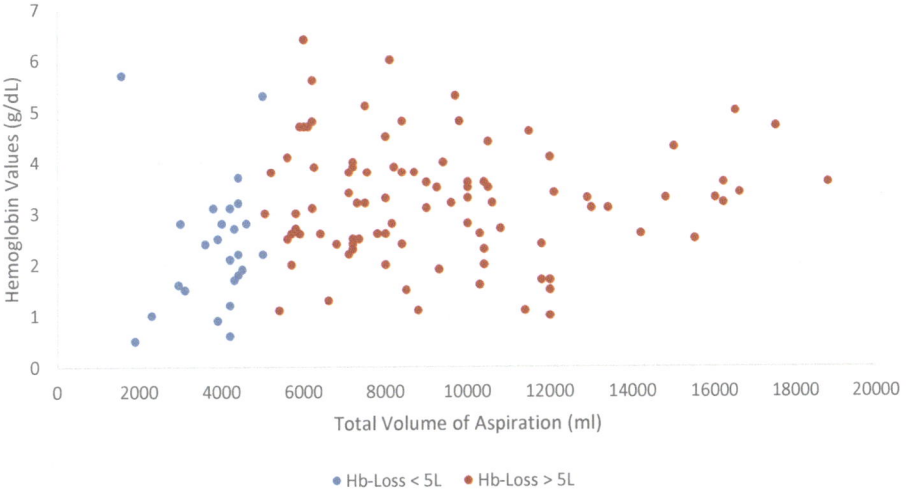

Figure 6. Scatter plot correlating hemoglobin loss to total volume of aspiration. A direct correlation can be seen within our study ($p = 0.012$). Women experiencing low-volume liposuction are displayed in blue; women experiencing high-volume liposuction are displayed in red.

BMI and duration of surgery still did not correlate significantly to hemoglobin loss ($p_{BMI} = 0.620$, $p_{duration} = 0.454$).

Investigating complication rates using the Clavien–Dindo Scale, no significant correlation could be seen regarding the duration of surgery ($p = 0.101$), age ($p = 0.116$), or BMI ($p = 0.143$). Also, no significant correlation could be seen between complication rates and the total volume of aspiration (0.176) (Table 7).

Table 7. Spearman Rho Rank analysis showing that the total volume of aspiration and complication rates do not correlate ($p = 0.176$).

		Spearman Rho Correlation Analysis		
			Complication Rates	Volume total Aspiration
Spearman Rho	Complication rates	Corr. Coefficient	1.000	0.124
		Sig. (2-tailed)		0.176
		N	121	121
	Volume total Aspiration	Corr. Coefficient	0.124	1.000
		Sig. (2-tailed)	0.176	
		N	121	121

Nonetheless, a statistical significance was seen between complication rates and hemoglobin loss ($p = 0.002$) (Table 8).

Table 8. Spearman Rho Rank analysis showing that postoperative complication rates significantly correlate to hemoglobin loss ($p = 0.002$).

		Spearman Rho Correlation Analysis		
			Complication rates	Hemoglobin Loss
Spearman Rho	Complication rates	Corr. Coefficient	1.000	0.275
		Sig. (2-tailed)		0.002
		N	121	121
	Hemoglobin Loss	Corr. Coefficient	0.275	1.000
		Sig. (2-tailed)	0.002	
		N	121	121

Postoperatively, 99 (81.82%) patients showed hemoglobin levels below 12 g/dL. In total, 101 (83.47%) patients did not show any kind of postoperative issues, while 20 (16.53%) patients did show complications, based on the Clavien–Dindo Classification. When performing independent t-tests, we observed a significant difference in hospital stay ($p = 0.012$) and duration of postoperative antithrombotic prophylaxis ($p = 0.05$) between patients with and without postoperative complications.

When comparing hemoglobin values and anemia, we also encountered statistical significances. Postoperative hemoglobin levels differed significantly between patients without and with postoperative complications ($p < 0.001$). Yet, preoperative hemoglobin values did not differ significantly ($p = 0.080$). Still, a tendency can be seen. The occurrence of anemia was additionally seen to be significantly different, both pre- ($p = 0.050$) and postoperatively ($p < 0.001$) (Table 9).

Conducting Spearman Rho correlation analyses, we additionally deciphered complications significantly correlating with hemoglobin values. Pre- ($p = 0.015$) and postoperative ($p < 0.001$) hemoglobin levels significantly correlated with the occurrence of postoperative complications. This was also true for hemoglobin loss ($p = 0.001$) and even the percentual difference in postoperative hemoglobin loss ($p < 0.001$). Further, preoperative anemia also correlated significantly with postoperative complication rates ($p < 0.001$). Still, postoperative anemia did not correlate significantly to higher complication rates ($p = 0.053$) (Table 10).

Table 9. Levene's Test of pre- and postoperative hemoglobin values and anemia compared between patients without and patients with postoperative complications. Here, a significant difference ($p < 0.001$) in postoperative hemoglobin values can be seen. Also, the occurrence of anemia, pre- ($p = 0.050$) and postoperatively ($p < 0.001$), showed statistical significance. Solely preoperative hemoglobin levels did not differ significantly ($p = 0.080$).

	Levene's Test of Equality of Variances						
	F	Sig.	T	df	One-sided p	Two-sided p	Mean difference
Hemoglobin preop	5.133	0.025	1.834	22.564	0.040	0.080	0.6128
Hemoglobin postop	3.463	0.065	5.195	119	<0.001	<0.001	1.4180
Anemia preop	42.321	<0.001	−2.078	20.487	0.025	0.050	−0.2104
Anemia postop	14.172	<0.001	−3.672	100	<0.001	<0.001	−0.1188

Table 10. Spearman Rho Rank analysis of complication rates in correlation to hemoglobin values preoperatively and postoperatively ($p_{preoperative} = 0.015$ and $p_{postoperative} < 0.001$), and anemia preoperatively and postoperatively ($p_{preoperative} =$ y 0.001 and $p_{postoperative} = 0.053$).

	Spearman Rho Correlation Analysis		
			Complication rates
Spearman Rho	Complication rates	Corr. Coefficient	1.000
		Sig. (2-tailed)	
		N	121
	Hemoglobin preop	Corr. Coefficient	−0.196
		Sig. (2-tailed)	0.015
		N	121
	Hemoglobin postop	Corr. Coefficient	−0.366
		Sig. (2-tailed)	<0.001
		N	121
	Anemia preop	Corr. Coefficient	0.298
		Sig. (2-tailed)	<0.001
		N	121
	Anemia postop	Corr. Coefficient	0.148
		Sig. (2-tailed)	0.053
		N	121

4. Discussion

Lipedema is an adipose tissue disorder mainly affecting women [10]. Since many patients show elevated BMI, high-volume reduction is often necessary [7,17]. This can either be achieved by performing several sessions of liposuction, or through less high-volume liposuction. Yet, multiple procedures entail higher costs for health care systems and patients, and require multiple applications of anesthesia, while only providing slow symptom relief [20]. Thus, high-volume liposuctions are more efficient and more patient-adapted [21–23]. Unfortunately, high-volume liposuctions have been condemned as risky procedures, as complication rates seem to increase with volume aspirated [24–26]. Nonetheless, liposuctions above this threshold are widely performed nowadays [16].

In our cohort, the mean total volume of aspiration was 8227.851 mL ± 3643.891 mL with a maximum of 18,800 mL in one session. However, our number of Class II complications of 3.31% did not exceed common rates described in the literature with a lower total volume aspirated [24]. Further, we did not see any significant difference in hospital stay, postoperative hemoglobin levels or overall complication rates between low- and high-volume liposuction sessions. Naturally, a significant difference in the duration of surgery and total volume of aspiration was apparent. Yet, these findings hold no clinical relevance, as a higher volume of aspiration requires more surgery time. Also, because our patients were divided into low- and high-volume liposuction groups, this result was expected. Still, the observed gap between the respective mean durations of surgery between our groups was not as significant as expected.

Among our patients, hemoglobin loss differed significantly ($p = 0.001$). Additionally, hemoglobin loss directly correlated with total volume of aspiration ($p = 0.012$). Interestingly, the total volume of aspiration did not correlate with complication rates ($p = 0.176$). As such, we assume that adverse events in high-volume liposuction are hemoglobin-dependent rather than volume-affiliated. Naturally, hemoglobin loss correlated directly with Class II complications ($p = 0.002$); nonetheless, this result was to be expected, as all patients experiencing Class II complications received blood transfusions.

These findings were also supported by the significant correlation between preoperative anemia and the presence of complications ($p < 0.001$), and the fact that women experiencing Class II complications showed preoperative anemia in 75% of cases. When stratifying patients based on the presence or absence of postoperative complications, those who experienced complications exhibited significantly lower perioperative hemoglobin levels compared to those without complications. Additionally, the incidence of postoperative anemia differed significantly between the groups. Correlating complication rates with hematologic parameters, we revealed significant associations with preoperative low hemoglobin levels ($p = 0.015$) and preoperative anemia ($p < 0.001$), but not with postoperative anemia ($p = 0.053$). These findings underscore the critical role of preoperative anemia as a pivotal factor in the development of postoperative complications. Finally, a direct correlation between complications and the duration of surgery could not be confirmed ($p = 0.101$). Neither could a longer duration of surgery be correlated to hemoglobin loss ($p = 0.454$).

Further, we identified preoperative anemia as a direct risk factor for postoperative complications in high-volume liposuction. This recognition was also seen in, e.g., anemic breast cancer patients experiencing higher drainage fluid volume after mastectomy [18], thus highlighting the key role of hemoglobin and its significance in postoperative sequelae. Therefore, lipedema patients should be evaluated precisely before surgery. As for the selective nature of high-volume liposuction, preoperative preparation is fundamental for patient safety [27].

Unfortunately, our study faces some limitations. Our department's focus on efficiently minimizing patients' pain may introduce a bias favoring high-volume liposuction. Further, the uneven distribution between groups poses a risk of distorting statistical analyses. Yet, as for the progressive nature of this disease, low-volume liposuctions are only seldomly encountered in our department. To more precisely address this important topic, prospective multicenter studies ought to be conducted, whereby the uneven patient distribution could be reduced. Further, long-term follow-ups need to be emphasized, to eradicate disruptive factors such as the under-reporting of possible complications after hospital discharge. Although none of our patients related such information, precise questioning could be implemented. Another limiting aspect could be the modified Klein's solution. The adding of adrenaline to our tumescence solution is intended to achieve vasoconstriction, which reduces bleeding and minimizes hemoglobin loss. Furthermore, the use of larger volumes of tumescence solution in high-volume liposuction may amplify this effect. Finally, the employment of bigger cannulas might also cause increased bleeding.

5. Conclusions

Our study highlights the significance of hemoglobin-dependency in complication rates of high-volume liposuction. Preoperatively anemic patients planned for high-volume liposuctions should be reconsidered or sufficiently prepared. Additionally, hematologic characteristics ought to be optimized, ahead of high-volume liposuction. By sustaining these features in high-volume liposuction, along with general perioperative security guidelines, this procedure can be improved upon in terms of feasibility and patient safety.

Author Contributions: Conceptualization, T.F., B.K., J.S., J.R., H.S., C.G., K.P., J.N., K.D.B. and K.F.S.; methodology, T.F., B.K., J.S., J.R., H.S., C.G., K.P., J.N., K.D.B. and K.F.S.; software, T.F., B.K., J.S., J.R., H.S., C.G., K.P., J.N., K.D.B. and K.F.S.; validation, T.F., B.K., J.S., J.R., H.S., C.G., K.P., J.N., K.D.B. and K.F.S.; formal analysis, T.F., B.K., J.S., J.R., H.S., C.G., K.P., J.N., K.D.B. and K.F.S.; resources, T.F., B.K., J.S., J.R., H.S., C.G., K.P., J.N., K.D.B. and K.F.S.; data curation, T.F., B.K., J.S., J.R., H.S., C.G., K.P., J.N., K.D.B. and K.F.S.; writing—original draft preparation, T.F., B.K., J.S., J.R., H.S., C.G., K.P., J.N., K.D.B. and K.F.S.; writing—review and editing, T.F., B.K., J.S., J.R., H.S., C.G., K.P., J.N., K.D.B. and K.F.S.; visualization, T.F., B.K., J.S., J.R., H.S., C.G., K.P., J.N., K.D.B. and K.F.S.; supervision, K.D.B. and K.F.S.; project administration, T.F., B.K., J.S., J.R., H.S., C.G., K.P., J.N., K.D.B. and K.F.S.; funding acquisition, T.F.; All authors have read and agreed to the published version of the manuscript.

Funding: This research received funding for open access publication by the Karl Landsteiner University of Health Sciences, Dr. Karl-Dorrek-Straße 30, 3500, Krems, Austria. The APC was funded by the Karl Landsteiner University of Health Sciences, Dr. Karl-Dorrek-Straße 30, 3500, Krems, Austria.

Institutional Review Board Statement: The study was conducted according to the guidelines of the Declaration of Helsinki and approved by the Institutional Ethics Committee of Karl Landsteiner University of Health Sciences Krems (protocol code: 1041/2021, 2 November 2021).

Informed Consent Statement: Patient consent was waived due to the retrospective character of this study.

Data Availability Statement: All the data analyzed during the current study are available from the corresponding author on reasonable request.

Acknowledgments: The authors want to appreciate the contribution of NÖ Landesgesundheitsagentur, legal entity of University Hospitals in Lower Austria, for providing the organizational framework to conduct this research. The authors also would like to acknowledge support by Open Access Publishing Fund of Karl Landsteiner University of Health Sciences, Krems, Austria.

Conflicts of Interest: The authors declare no conflicts of interest.

References

1. Amato, A.C.; Amato, J.L.; Benitti, D. Efficacy of Liposuction in the Treatment of Lipedema: A Meta-Analysis. *Cureus* **2024**, *16*, e55260. [CrossRef] [PubMed]
2. Okhovat, J.P.; Alavi, A. Lipedema: A Review of the Literature. *Int. J. Low. Extrem. Wounds* **2015**, *14*, 262–267. [CrossRef] [PubMed]
3. Buso, G.; Depairon, M.; Tomson, D.; Raffoul, W.; Vettor, R.; Mazzolai, L. Lipedema: A Call to Action! *Obesity* **2019**, *27*, 1567–1576. [CrossRef] [PubMed]
4. Herbst, K.L.; Kahn, L.A.; Iker, E.; Ehrlich, C.; Wright, T.; McHutchison, L.; Schwartz, J.; Sleigh, M.; Donahue, P.M.; Lisson, K.H.; et al. Standard of care for lipedema in the United States. *Phlebology* **2021**, *36*, 779–796. [CrossRef]
5. Wold, L.E.; Hines, E.A., Jr.; Allen, E.V. Lipedema of the legs; a syndrome characterized by fat legs and edema. *Ann. Intern. Med.* **1951**, *34*, 1243–1250. [CrossRef]
6. Child, A.H.; Gordon, K.D.; Sharpe, P.; Brice, G.; Ostergaard, P.; Jeffery, S.; Mortimer, P.S. Lipedema: An inherited condition. *Am. J. Med. Genet. A* **2010**, *152A*, 970–976. [CrossRef]
7. Flores, T.; Kerschbaumer, C.; Jaklin, F.J.; Glisic, C.; Sabitzer, H.; Nedomansky, J.; Wolf, P.; Weber, M.; Bergmeister, K.D.; Schrogendorfer, K.F. High-Volume Liposuction in Lipedema Patients: Effects on Serum Vitamin D. *J. Clin. Med.* **2024**, *13*, 2846. [CrossRef]
8. Bauer, A.T.; von Lukowicz, D.; Lossagk, K.; Aitzetmueller, M.; Moog, P.; Cerny, M.; Erne, H.; Schmauss, D.; Duscher, D.; Machens, H.G. New Insights on Lipedema: The Enigmatic Disease of the Peripheral Fat. *Plast. Reconstr. Surg.* **2019**, *144*, 1475–1484. [CrossRef]
9. Schmeller, W.; Meier-Vollrath, I. Tumescent liposuction: A new and successful therapy for lipedema. *J. Cutan. Med. Surg.* **2006**, *10*, 7–10. [CrossRef]
10. Poojari, A.; Dev, K.; Rabiee, A. Lipedema: Insights into Morphology, Pathophysiology, and Challenges. *Biomedicines* **2022**, *10*, 3081. [CrossRef]
11. Wollina, U. Lipedema-An update. *Dermatol. Ther.* **2019**, *32*, e12805. [CrossRef] [PubMed]

12. Pajula, S.; Jyranki, J.; Tukiainen, E.; Koljonen, V. Complications after lower body contouring surgery due to massive weight loss unaffected by weight loss method. *J. Plast. Reconstr. Aesthet. Surg.* **2019**, *72*, 649–655. [CrossRef] [PubMed]
13. Herbst, K.L. Subcutaneous Adipose Tissue Diseases: Dercum Disease, Lipedema, Familial Multiple Lipomatosis, and Madelung Disease. In *Endotext*; Feingold, K.R., Anawalt, B., Blackman, M.R., Boyce, A., Chrousos, G., Corpas, E., de Herder, W.W., Dhatariya, K., Dungan, K., Hofland, J., et al., Eds.; MDText.com, Inc.: South Dartmouth, MA, USA, 2000.
14. Keith, L.; Seo, C.A.; Rowsemitt, C.; Pfeffer, M.; Wahi, M.; Staggs, M.; Dudek, J.; Gower, B.; Carmody, M. Ketogenic diet as a potential intervention for lipedema. *Med. Hypotheses* **2021**, *146*, 110435. [CrossRef] [PubMed]
15. Iverson, R.E.; Lynch, D.J.; American Society of Plastic Surgeons Committee on Patient. Practice advisory on liposuction. *Plast. Reconstr. Surg.* **2004**, *113*, 1478–1490; discussion 1491–1475. [CrossRef]
16. Mortada, H.; Alshenaifi, S.A.; Samawi, H.A.; Marzoug, M.M.; Alhumsi, T.; Alaithan, B. The Safety of Large-Amount Liposuction: A Retrospective Analysis of 28 Cases. *J. Cutan. Aesthet. Surg.* **2023**, *16*, 227–231. [CrossRef]
17. Golpanian, S.; Rahal, G.A.; Rahal, W.J. Outpatient-Based High-Volume Liposuction: A Retrospective Review of 310 Consecutive Patients. *Aesthet. Surg. J.* **2023**, *43*, 1310–1324. [CrossRef]
18. Flores, T.; Jaklin, F.J.; Rohrbacher, A.; Schrogendorfer, K.F.; Bergmeister, K.D. Perioperative Risk Factors for Prolonged Blood Loss and Drainage Fluid Secretion after Breast Reconstruction. *J. Clin. Med.* **2022**, *11*, 808. [CrossRef]
19. WHO. *Obesity*; WHO: Geneva, Switzerland, 2023.
20. Forner-Cordero, I.; Forner-Cordero, A.; Szolnoky, G. Update in the management of lipedema. *Int. Angiol.* **2021**, *40*, 345–357. [CrossRef]
21. Taha, A.A.; Tahseen, H. Liposuction: Keeping It Safe! *Plast. Reconstr. Surg. Glob. Open* **2020**, *8*, e2783. [CrossRef]
22. Bellini, E.; Grieco, M.P.; Raposio, E. A journey through liposuction and liposculture: Review. *Ann. Med. Surg.* **2017**, *24*, 53–60. [CrossRef]
23. Tabbal, G.N.; Ahmad, J.; Lista, F.; Rohrich, R.J. Advances in liposuction: Five key principles with emphasis on patient safety and outcomes. *Plast. Reconstr. Surg. Glob. Open* **2013**, *1*, e75. [CrossRef] [PubMed]
24. Cardenas-Camarena, L.; Andres Gerardo, L.P.; Duran, H.; Bayter-Marin, J.E. Strategies for Reducing Fatal Complications in Liposuction. *Plast. Reconstr. Surg. Glob. Open* **2017**, *5*, e1539. [CrossRef] [PubMed]
25. Dixit, V.V.; Wagh, M.S. Unfavourable outcomes of liposuction and their management. *Indian. J. Plast. Surg.* **2013**, *46*, 377–392. [CrossRef] [PubMed]
26. Saleh, Y.; El-Oteify, M.; Abd-El-Salam, A.E.; Tohamy, A.; Abd-Elsayed, A.A. Safety and benefits of large-volume liposuction: A single center experience. *Int. Arch. Med.* **2009**, *2*, 4. [CrossRef] [PubMed]
27. Lamperti, M.; Romero, C.S.; Guarracino, F.; Cammarota, G.; Vetrugno, L.; Tufegdzic, B.; Lozsan, F.; Macias Frias, J.J.; Duma, A.; Bock, M.; et al. Preoperative assessment of adults undergoing elective noncardiac surgery: Updated guidelines from the European Society of Anaesthesiology and Intensive Care. *Eur. J. Anaesthesiol.* **2025**, *42*, 1–35. [CrossRef]

Disclaimer/Publisher's Note: The statements, opinions and data contained in all publications are solely those of the individual author(s) and contributor(s) and not of MDPI and/or the editor(s). MDPI and/or the editor(s) disclaim responsibility for any injury to people or property resulting from any ideas, methods, instructions or products referred to in the content.

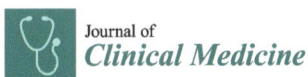

Article

Paravertebral Blocks in Implant-Based Breast Reconstruction Do Not Induce Increased Postoperative Blood or Drainage Fluid Loss

Tonatiuh Flores [1,2,*], Florian J. Jaklin [3], Martin S. Mayrl [1], Celina Kerschbaumer [1], Christina Glisic [1,2], Kristina Pfoser [1,2], David B. Lumenta [4], Klaus F. Schrögendorfer [1,2], Christoph Hörmann [1,5] and Konstantin D. Bergmeister [1,2,3]

1. Karl Landsteiner University of Health Sciences, Dr-Karl-Dorrek-Straße 30, 3500 Krems, Austria; celina.kerschbaumer@outlook.com (C.K.); christina.glisic@stpoelten.lknoe.at (C.G.); kristina.pfoser@stpoelten.lknoe.at (K.P.); klaus.schroegendorfer@stpoelten.lknoe.at (K.F.S.); christop.hoerman@stpoelten.lknoe.at (C.H.); konstantin.bergmeister@stpoelten.lknoe.at (K.D.B.)
2. Clinical Department of Plastic, Aesthetic and Reconstructive Surgery, University Clinic of St. Poelten, 3100 St. Poelten, Austria
3. Clinical Laboratory for Bionic Extremity Reconstruction, University Clinic for Plastic, Reconstructive and Aesthetic Surgery, Medical University of Vienna, 1090 Vienna, Austria; florian.jaklin@meduniwien.ac.at
4. Division of Plastic, Aesthetic and Reconstructive Surgery, Department of Surgery, Medical University of Graz, 8010 Graz, Austria
5. Clinical Department of Anesthesiology and Intensive Care Medicine, University Clinic of St. Poelten, 3100 St. Poelten, Austria
* Correspondence: tonatiuh.flores@stpoelten.lknoe.at; Tel.: +43-2742-9004-23624

Abstract: Background: Women undergoing a mastectomy often suffer severely from the sequelae of losing one or both breasts. Implant-based breast reconstruction restores female body integrity but can result in significant postoperative pain. The use of paravertebral catheters has been shown to aid significantly in pain management during the postoperative recovery. However, the vasodilation that is induced by paravertebral blocks may lead to prolonged drainage fluid secretion, blood loss and increased likelihood of revision surgery. Therefore, we analyzed the effects of paravertebral blocks after combined mastectomy and immediate breast reconstruction. **Methods**: We analyzed 115 breast surgeries at the department of Plastic Surgery at the University clinic of St. Poelten between 1 August 2018 and 31 December 2022. Patients were analyzed regarding postoperative hemoglobin loss and drainage fluid volumes and their correlation with paravertebral blocks. Statistical analyses were performed using Levene's Test for Equality of Variances within our cohort. **Results**: The postoperative hemoglobin loss did not differ significantly between our groups ($p = 0.295$). Furthermore, a paravertebral block did not increase the amount of postoperative drainage fluid volumes ($p = 0.508$). Women receiving paravertebral blocks also did not stay longer in hospitals ($p = 0.276$). No paravertebral block-associated complication was seen. **Conclusions**: In this study, we demonstrated paravertebral blocks to be safe adjuncts in breast reconstruction to minimize pain without leading to increased blood loss or seroma formation. This indicated that vasodilatation induced by paravertebral blocks did not negatively influence the postoperative recovery. In conclusion, postoperative pain management using paravertebral blocks can be a beneficial therapeutic adjunct in surgical management of breast cancer patients.

Keywords: breast cancer; breast reconstruction; pain catheter; postoperative blood loss; drainage volume; patient after-care

1. Introduction

Mastectomy due to breast cancer severely impacts the well-being of affected women on account of a loss of body integrity [1–5]. Consequently, breast reconstruction represents an essential pillar of modern breast cancer treatment to reduce the suffering of breast cancer patients [6–9]. During surgery, the primary goal is complete tumor resection, and thus, the residual skin often experiences severe perfusion disturbances, which can negatively affect the direct implant insertion [10–15]. Here, submuscular expanders help to generate sufficient soft tissue for further reconstruction without stressing the residual skin [16–18]. However, their placement entails painful muscle stretching, leading to postoperative discomfort and pain [19–22].

Since the introduction of paravertebral catheters, postoperative pain has decreased noticeably for women after a mastectomy [23–27]. Its popularity has increased over the past decades and is now part of the advanced perioperative armamentarium after mastectomy [26,28,29]. Yet, paravertebral blocks (PVBs) are associated with several undesired issues [30–34]. Pneumothorax, as its most commonly encountered complication, dislocation and occlusion are frequently seen [30–32,34]. And while the numbing of pain receptors is the primary goal, vasodilation is simultaneously provoked due to the sympathicolysis [35]. Whilst vasodilatation is a desired effect in replantation surgery, it may result in prolonged bleeding or an increased postoperative drainage fluid volume and thus lead to complications [36–39].

In this paper, we analyzed the effect of paravertebral blocks on the postoperative blood loss and drainage fluid volume in women undergoing breast reconstruction after mastectomy. Our aim was to investigate the impact of vasodilation on the postoperative hemoglobin levels and drainage fluid volumes. To our knowledge, this is the first study investigating the effect of paravertebral catheters on breast cancer patients after mastectomy.

2. Materials and Methods

2.1. Study Design and Patient Analysis

In this study, we analyzed patients undergoing subcutaneous mastectomy and consecutive breast reconstruction at the Clinical Department for Plastic, Aesthetic and Reconstructive Surgery at the University Hospital St. Poelten between 1 August 2018 and 31 December 2022. This study was conducted as a retrospective single-center study. Ethical approval was obtained from the local institutional review board at the Karl Landsteiner University of Health Sciences Krems (reference number: ECS 1085/2023). Analyzed factors included the patients' age at surgery, BMI, mastectomy weight, mastectomy side (unilateral, bilateral), sentinel lymph node dissection, axillary dissection, perioperative hemoglobin and hematocrit, postoperative drainage fluid volume, operation time and duration of hospital stay.

Hemoglobin values (g/dL) were analyzed prior to surgery and on the first postoperative day. Anemia was defined as values below 12 g/dL according to the WHO classification [39]. The drainage output was documented every 12 h until the removal of the drainage catheters. Drainage removal was conducted if the output was less than 30 mL in 24 h. The patients included were divided into two groups, based on whether they were receiving paravertebral block (paravertebral block (PVB) group) or not (non-paravertebral block (non-PVB) group). Every patient at our department was offered PVB. Women accepting and then receiving PVB were added to the PVB group. In case of PVB rejection by patients, PVB was not installed. Thus, patients were transferred to the non-PVB group.

None of the included patients displayed any kind of liver abnormalities, hematopoietic disorders, or diseases in need of immunomodulatory medication. Further, neoadjuvant chemo-, radiation- and hormone therapies were analyzed in terms of their influence on blood loss or drainage fluid volume in this study.

2.2. Paravertebral Block

Every patient at our department who was scheduled for mastectomy was offered a paravertebral block for adequate and facilitated postoperative pain management. The procedure was ultrasound-guided and performed under sterile conditions on the day before surgery by an anesthesiologist who is specifically trained for this intervention. The installation of the paravertebral catheters was conducted either with the patient sitting or in a lateral decubitus position at the level of Th 4. After successful installation, continuity testing was performed with two milliliters of Ropivacain (Ropinaest®, Gebro Pharma, Bahnhofbichl 11, 6391 Fieberbrunn, Germany) (Figure 1). The PVB cable was fixed with transparent occlusion foil to be able to fully review the catheter at least once a day and to prevent unintentional dislocation.

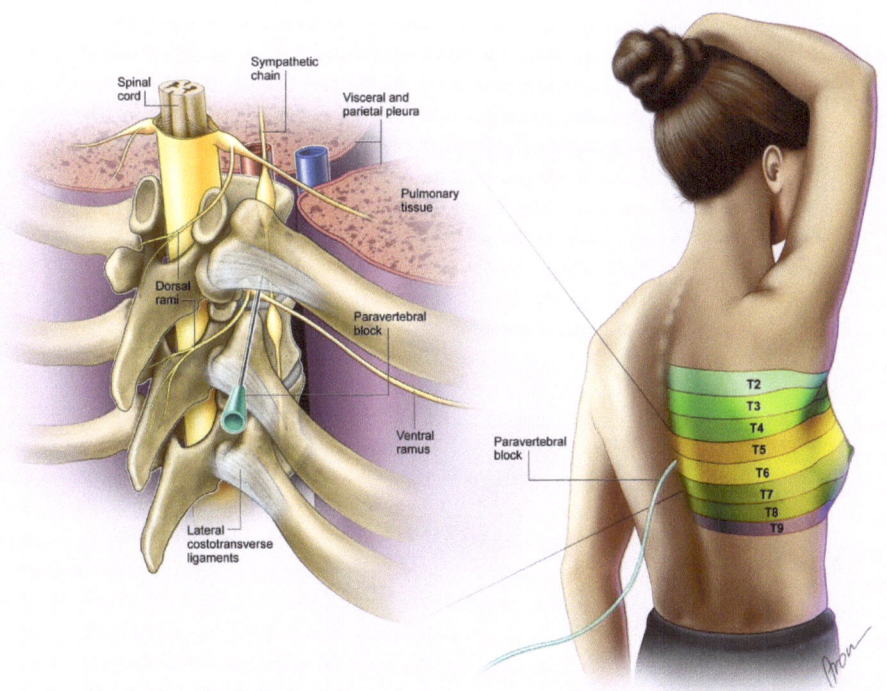

Figure 1. PVB in place blocking the respective dermatomes for sufficient pain relief after mastectomy. Note the proximity of the catheter to the sympathetic chain. The segments T2–T9 indicate sensory innervated dermatomes.

Additionally, a chest X-ray was performed for pneumothorax exclusion. Each catheter was connected to an ON-Q® pump (On-Q® pain relief system, AVANOS Medical, c/o Pier 11, Schauenburgerstraße 10, 20095 Hamburg, Germany) with a select-a-flow variable rate controller with a reservoir of 400 mL, containing Ropivacain. The dosage settings were at 2, 4, 6, 8, 10, 12 or 14 mL/h, individually adjusted to the patient's pain level. Each paravertebral catheter was injected with two milliliters of Ropivacain (Ropinaest®, Gebro Pharma 6391 Fieberbrunn, Germany) 30 min before the incision.

Catheters were reduced starting on the second postoperative day by 2 mL/h each day until reaching 0 mL/h. The standard postoperative dosage for postoperative catheter influx was 10 mL/h. PVBs were checked by anesthesiologists daily until removal.

2.3. Operative Procedure

Subcutaneous mastectomies were conducted either through lateral incision or in case of a simultaneous reduction via inverted T incision. A retromammillary cylinder was additionally retrieved and sent for frozen section examination to determine whether the NAC (nipple areolar complex) had to be removed or not. If the sentinel lymph node tested positive intraoperatively, axillary dissection was performed after the mastectomy. If the retromammillary cylinder tested positive intraoperatively, the NAC was removed.

In case of sufficient subcutaneous tissue, immediate prepectoral breast reconstruction, using Mentor implants (MENTOR® Contour Profile Gel™ (CPG™), Mentor Worldwide LLC, 31 Technology Drive, Suite 200, Irvine, CA 92618, USA) with a textured surface and Serasynth® Mesh (Serag-Wiessner GmbH & Co. Kg Zum Kugelfang 8–12, 95119 Naila, Germany), was performed.

If the subcutaneous layers did not seem resilient enough for prepectoral implant placing, submuscular tissue expanders were installed. All implants had textured and anatomical properties (Mentor Siltex® Contour Profile™ Becker™ 35 Expander, Mentor Worldwide LLC, 31 Technology Drive, Suite 200, Irvine, CA 92618, USA). Submuscular pocket preparation was performed through incising the major pectoral muscle parallel to its muscle fiber course, approximately at the level of the fourth to fifth intercostal space. The serratus anterior fascia was partially raised to support the implant inferiorly and laterally if needed. Port systems were installed at the level of the anterior axillary line at the level of Th 5. If no axillary dissection was performed, subcutaneous and submuscular drains were placed. In case of axillary dissection, one additional drain was inserted in the axillary wound cavity. Drains were removed in case of less than 30 mL of fluid within 24 h.

2.4. Statistics and Data Management

The endpoint of our analyses was to assess the hemoglobin loss and the volume of the postoperative drainage fluid after mastectomy. Our dataset was divided into two groups: women with and women without paravertebral block. All data were reported anonymously. The data protection management complied with Austrian legislation. Data collection and processing were performed with Microsoft Excel (Microsoft corp., Washington, DC, USA), and statistical analyses were performed using IBM SPSS Statistics version 29 (©IBM, Armonk, NY, USA). Nominal data are described using absolute frequencies and percentages. For metric data, the mean and standard deviation are indicated. To correlate the amount of postoperative drainage fluid volume and hemoglobin loss to paravertebral blocks, correlation analyses using independent samples Mann–Whitney U Tests were performed. Further, paired t-test analyses were conducted to compare groups, specifically regarding the postoperative drainage volumes of patients with and without paravertebral block. A two-sided $p \leq 0.05$ was regarded as statistically significant.

3. Results

In total, 1128 breast surgeries were analyzed within this study. Of these, 432 were excluded due to being body forming surgeries, 119 due to being breast implant revisions, 142 due to being second-stage reconstruction, 215 due to being non-implant-based cancer-related breast surgeries, and 3 due to being sole tissue expander implantations. Additionally, 65 surgeries had to be excluded due to a lack of sufficient data. Finally, 152 mastectomies in 115 patients with consecutive breast reconstruction met our criteria and were included in this study.

Here, 124 tissue expanders and 28 definitive breast implants were implanted in 115 patients. In our study group, 52 (45.22%) women received preoperative paravertebral catheter, and 63 (54.78%) underwent surgery without paravertebral block (Table 1).

Table 1. Demography of patients included in this study.

Patient Characteristics		Without PVB	With PVB	Overall Patients	p-Values
Number		63 (54.78%)	52 (45.22%)	115	
Age (years)	Mean	46.77	48.37	47.5	0.438
	Min–Max	23–76	29–70	23–76	
	STD	±11.08	±10.54	±10.82	
BMI (kg/m^2)	Mean	25.40	24.16	24.84	0.152
	Min–Max	16.4–41.1	17.9–37.5	16.4–41.1	
	STD	±4.58	±4.46	±4.59	
Duration of surgery (min)	Mean	181.81	168.56	175.82	0.150
	Min–Max	85–329	95–264	85–329	
	STD	±53.02	±41.97	48.79	
Number of inserted implants	Total	87 (57.24%)	65 (42.76%)	152	0.133
	Expanders	68 (78.16%)	56 (86.15%)	124 (81.49%)	
	Def. Implants	19 (21.84%)	9 (13.85%)	28 (18.41%)	
Hospital stay (days)	Mean	8.87	8.52	8.71	0.396
	Min–Max	4–18	5–15	4–18	
	STD	±2.30	±2.07	±2.21	
Mastectomies total		87 (57.24%)	65 (42.76%)	152	0.204
Sentinel lymph node	Total	39 (50%)	39 (50%)	78	0.234
Axillary dissection	Total	24 (66.67%)	12 (33.33%)	36	0.104
Hb pre-op (g/dL)	Mean	13.14	12.92	13.04	0.404
	Min–Max	9.8–16.2	9.9–14.9	9.8–16.2	
	STD	±1.40	±1.30	±1.37	
Hb post-op (g/dL)	Mean	10.42	10.41	10.49	0.615
	Min–Max	7–10.3	10.2–11.8	7–11.8	
	STD	±1.41	±1.38	±1.71	
Hb Difference pre-post	Mean	−2.71	−2.52	−2.55	0.856
	Min–Max	−5.9–+7.1	−5.6–+0.3	+0.3–−5.9	
	STD	±1.31	±1.16	±1.54	
Drainage volume (mL)	Mean	1053.02	962.21	997	0.323
	Min–Max	300–2530	285–2380	285–2530	
	STD	±508.21	±453.96	±496.39	
Drainage inlay time (d)	Mean	7.38	7.25	7.32	0.957
	Min–Max	3–11	4–14	3–14	
	STD	±1.91	±1.95	±1.93	

3.1. Patient Demographics

The mean overall patient age at surgery was 47.50 years ± 10.82 years, ranging from 23 to 76 years (Table 1). The mean BMI was 28.84 kg/m^2 ± 4.59 kg/m^2, ranging from 16.4 to 41.1 kg/m^2. The mean duration of surgery was 175.82 min ± 48.79 min, varying from 85 to 329 min. The mean hospital stay was 8.71 days ± 2.21 days, ranging from 4 to 18 days.

The mean total mastectomy weight was 636.32 ± 415.48 g, ranging from 285 to 2543 g. The mean unilateral mastectomy weight on the left side was 319.59 ± 329.30 g, with a minimum weight of 84 g and a maximum weight of 1805 g. The mean unilateral mastectomy weight on the right side was 316.73 ± 318.12 g, ranging from 70 to 1286 g in total. Women without PVB experienced bilateral mastectomy in 24 (27.59%) cases and women with PVB in 13 (20.97%) cases. Overall, 78 (67.83%) patients underwent sentinel lymph node dissection. In addition, 64 (82.05%) were unilateral, and 7 (17.95%) were bilateral. A total of 36 (31.30%) patients received axillary dissection. Of these, 16 (44.44%) were left-sided, 18 (50%) were right-sided, and 1 (5.56%) was bilateral.

The mean overall Hb loss was 2.55 ± 1.54 g/dL (Table 1). Preoperative anemia was seen in 28 (33.05%) of our patients. The mean preoperative Hb levels were 13.04 g/dL ± 1.37 g/dL. Postoperatively, 100 (86.96%) patients showed hemoglobin levels below 12 g/dL. The mean postoperative Hb levels were 10.49 ±1.71 g/dL overall.

3.1.1. Non-PVB Group

In total, 63 (54.78%) patients were included in this group. The mean patient age at surgery was 46.77 years ± 11.08 years. In this group, 87 (57.24%) mastectomies were performed. Consecutively, 68 (78.16%) tissue expanders and 19 (21.84%) definitive breast implants were installed. The mean Hb loss was 2.71 ± 1.31 g/dL. The mean drainage fluid volume was 1053.02 ± 508.21 mL (Figure 2).

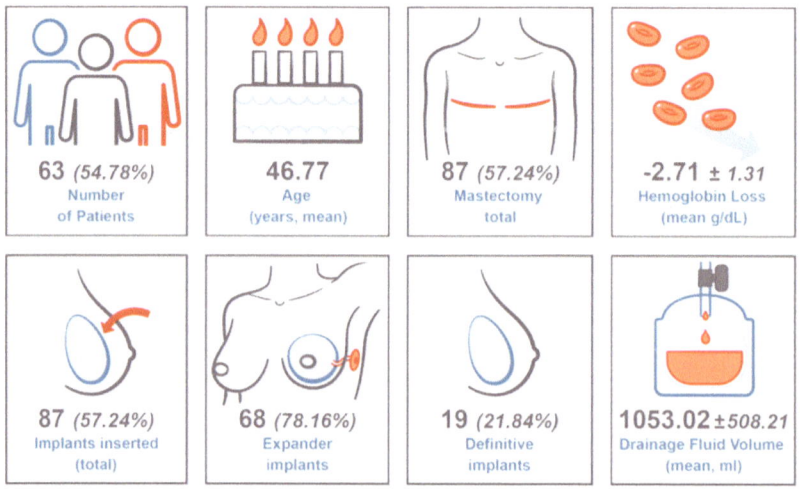

Figure 2. Key data chart for included patients without paravertebral block (PVB) and clinical findings.

In total, 23 (36.51%) women received neoadjuvant chemotherapy, 7 (11.11%) underwent neoadjuvant radiation therapy, and none had neoadjuvant hormone therapy.

3.1.2. PVB Group

In total, 52 (45.22%) patients were included in this group. The mean patient age at surgery was 48.37 years ± 10.54 years. In this group, 65 (42.76%) mastectomies were performed. Consecutively, 56 (86.15%) tissue expanders and 9 (13.85%) definitive breast implants were installed. The mean Hb loss was 2.52 ± 1.16 g/dL. The mean drainage fluid volume was 962.21 ± 453.96 mL (Figure 3).

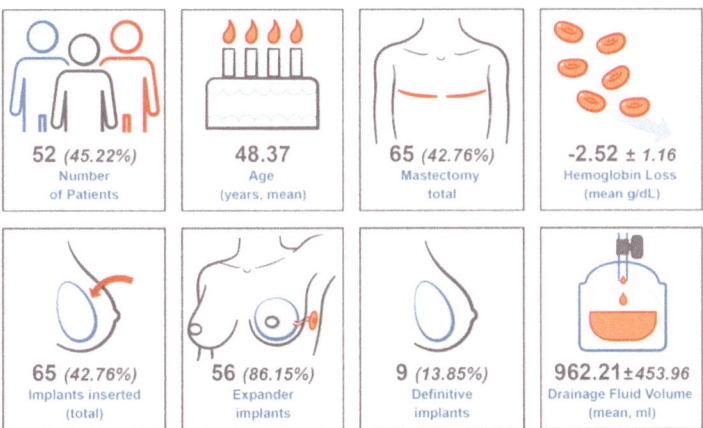

Figure 3. Key data chart for included PVB patients and clinical findings.

In total, 21 (40.38%) women received neoadjuvant chemotherapy, 4 (7.7%) underwent neoadjuvant radiation therapy, and none had neoadjuvant hormone therapy.

3.2. Hemoglobin Levels

The hemoglobin levels did not differ significantly between the groups. The mean preoperative Hb level in women without PVB was 13.14 ± 1.40 g/dL. Women with PVB showed a mean preoperative Hb level of 12.92 ± 1.30 g/dL (Figure 4). Postoperatively, no significant difference was seen either, as the mean postoperative Hb was 10.42 ± 1.41 g/dL in the non-PVB group and 10.41 ± 1.38 g/dL in the PVB group (Figure 4).

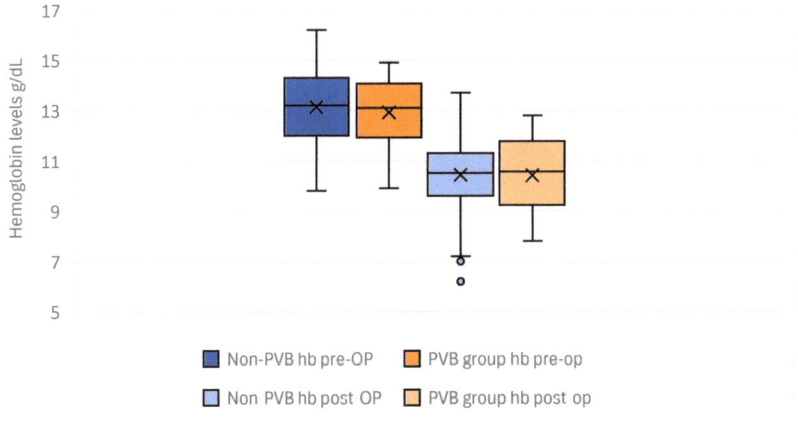

Figure 4. Boxplot of the hemoglobin levels of the groups. The preoperative values can be seen on the left in darker colors (dark blue: non-PVB group; dark orange: PVB group). The postoperative hemoglobin levels can be seen on the right in brighter colors (light blue: non-PVB group; light orange: PVB group). Although a clear difference in pre- and postoperative values is shown, no statistical significance could be proven. Outliers are depicted as dots.

Conducting a *T*-Test for the Equality of Means, no significant difference was found between the preoperative and postoperative hemoglobin levels between our groups ($p_{preoperative}$ = 0.404; $p_{postoperative}$ = 0.615) (Table 2).

Table 2. *T*-Test for Equality of Means regarding hemoglobin difference between our groups, preoperatively and postoperatively. Our analyses showed no significant difference between the pre- and postoperative hemoglobin levels of the groups ($p_{preoperative}$ = 0.404; $p_{postoperative}$ = 0.615).

	T-Test for Equality of Means						
	F	Sig.	T	df	One-Sided *p*	Two-Sided *p*	Mean Difference
Hemoglobin preoperative	0.087	0.769	0.838	113	0.202	**0.404**	0.2151
Hemoglobin postoperative	0.026	0.873	0.504	113	0.308	**0.615**	0.1624
			0.520	110.990	302	0.604	0.1624

The mean Hb loss was 2.71 ± 1.31 g/dL in the non-PVB group and 2.52 ± 1.16 g/dL in the PVB group (Figure 5).

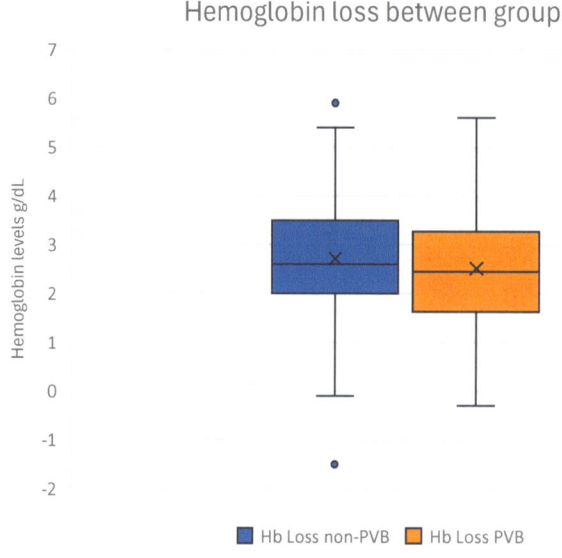

Figure 5. Boxplot of hemoglobin losses of groups. Non-paravertebral block patients can be seen on the left, and patients with paravertebral block are depicted on the right. No statistical significance can be seen in the difference in hemoglobin drop between the groups. Outliers are displayed as dots.

The *T*-Test for Equality of Means showed no statistical significance in Hb loss between our groups (p = 0.295) (Table 3).

Table 3. *T*-Test for Equality of Means showing no significance in the difference between pre- and postoperative hemoglobin values (*p* = 0.295). This shows that sympathicolysis makes no significant contribution to the postoperative hemoglobin loss.

	T-Test for Equality of Means						
	F	Sig.	T	df	One-Sided *p*	Two-Sided *p*	Mean Difference
Hemoglobin Loss	0.135	0.714	1.045	115	0.149	**0.295**	0.243

Correlating the influence of PVB on the postoperative Hb loss, no statistical difference could be observed (*p* = 0.397), demonstrating that paravertebral catheters had no significant impact on the perioperative hemoglobin loss within our cohort.

3.3. Drainage Fluid Volume

The mean drainage fluid volume was 1053.02 ± 508.21 mL in patients without paravertebral block and 962.21 ± 453.96 mL in women with paravertebral block (Figure 6).

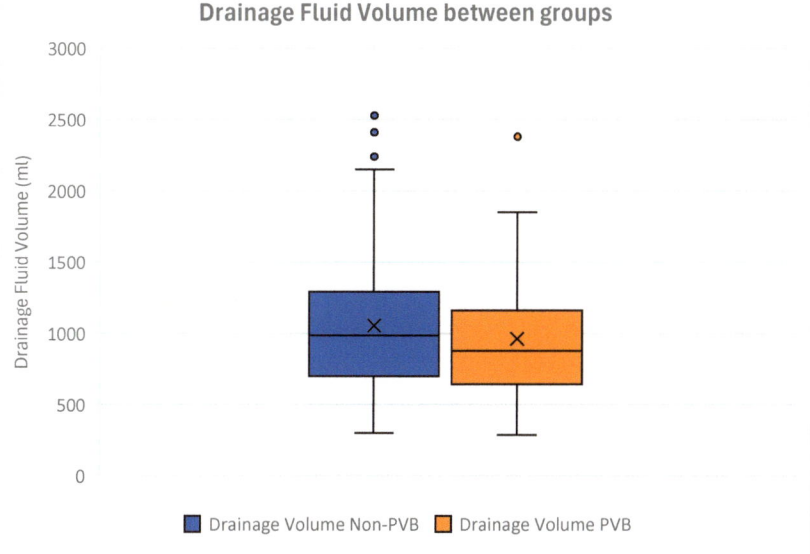

Figure 6. Boxplot showing the drainage fluid volumes of the groups. Non-paravertebral block patients can be seen on the left, while patients with paravertebral block are depicted on the right. No significant difference can be observed between the groups regarding postoperative drainage fluid loss. Outliers are displayed as dots.

The *T*-Test for Equality of Means displayed no statistical difference between the postoperative drainage fluid volumes (*p* = 0.508) (Table 4).

Table 4. *T*-testing of independent samples showing no significant difference in postoperative drainage fluid volumes between women with and without paravertebral block ($p = 0.508$). This demonstrates that postoperative drainage fluid volumes are not affected by paravertebral catheters and consecutive sympathicolysis.

	T-Test for Equality of Means						
	F	Sig.	T	df	One-Sided p	Two-Sided p	Mean Difference
Drainage fluid volume	0.388	0.543	0.665	115	0.254	**0.508**	61.788

Conducting independent samples analyses, no significant influence of PVB on the postoperative drainage fluid volume could be seen ($p = 0.367$), demonstrating that the drainage fluid volume was not affected by paravertebral catheters.

3.4. Duration of Surgery

Women without paravertebral block showed a mean surgery time of 181.81 ± 53.02 min. The mean duration of surgery was 168.56 ± 41.97 min in patients with PVB (Figure 7).

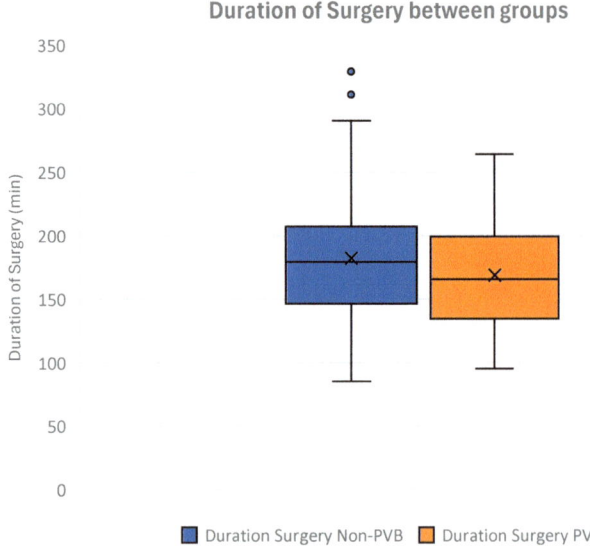

Figure 7. Boxplot of the durations of surgery of the groups. Women without paravertebral block experienced longer operation times. Non-paravertebral block patients can be seen on the left (blue), while patients with paravertebral block are depicted on the right (orange). Outliers are displayed as dots.

Our analyses displayed no significant difference regarding the duration of surgery between our groups. By conducting a *T*-Test for Equality of Means, this was statistically proven ($p = 0.150$) (Table 5).

Table 5. *T*-Test for Equality of Means demonstrating no statistical significance in the duration of surgery between the groups (*p* = 0.150).

	T-Test for Equality of Means						
	F	Sig.	T	df	One-Sided *p*	Two-Sided *p*	Mean Difference
Duration of Surgery	0.682	0.411	1.450	113	0.075	**0.150**	13.251

Analyzing the correlation of paravertebral blocks and the duration of surgery, no statistical significance could be seen (*p* = 0.260). This indicated that women receiving paravertebral blocks did not experience a longer duration of surgery than women without paravertebral block.

3.5. Hospital Stay

Women without paravertebral catheters showed a mean in-hospital duration of 8.87 days ± 2.30, whereas women with paravertebral block stayed in hospital for a mean of 8.52 days ± 2.07 (Figure 8).

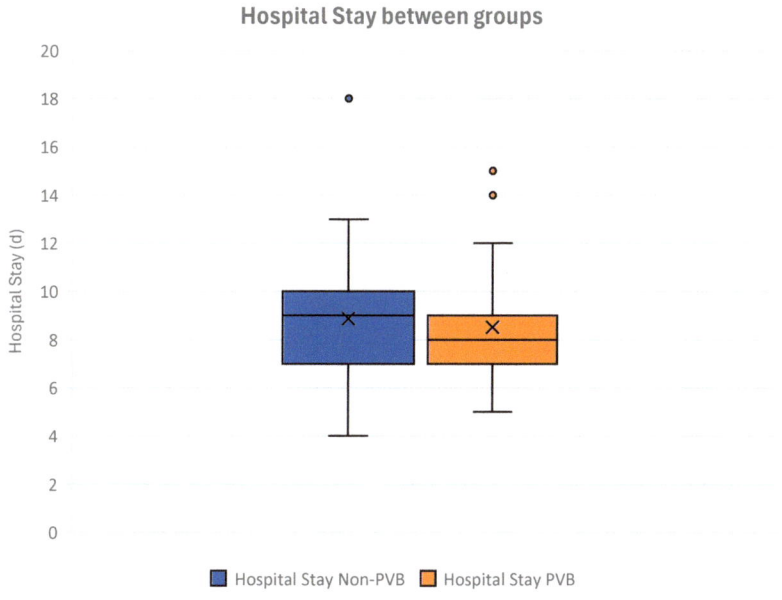

Figure 8. Boxplot of the lengths of hospital stay of the groups. Non-paravertebral block patients can be seen on the left, while patients with paravertebral block are depicted on the right. The duration of in-hospital stay did not differ significantly between groups. Outliers can be seen as dots.

Our analyses showed no statistical significance in the duration of hospital stay between women with and without paravertebral catheters (*p* = 0.348) (Table 6).

Table 6. Independent sample T-testing of lengths of hospital stay of both groups. Here, no statistical significance between the in-hospital duration can be observed ($p = 0.348$). This shows that women with or without PVB were admitted for a similar time-period.

	T-Test for Equality of Means						
	F	Sig.	T	df	One-Sided p	Two-Sided p	Mean Difference
Hospital stay	0.823	0.366	0.947	115	0.173	**0.348**	0.388

Further, no statistical significance between our groups could be seen after performing correlation analyses ($p = 0.275$). This showed that paravertebral block had no influence on the duration of hospital stay.

3.6. Neoadjuvant Breast Cancer-Related Therapy

Women without PVB had neoadjuvant chemotherapy in 23 (36.51%) cases, whereas patients receiving PVB underwent neoadjuvant chemotherapy in 21 cases (40.38%).

Neoadjuvant radiation therapy was performed in 7 (11.11%) cases in the non-PVB group and in 4 (7.7%) case in the PVB group. Performing independent *t*-testing, no statistical significance could be observed, neither in neoadjuvant chemotherapy ($p = 0.674$) or radiation therapy ($p = 0.229$).

Conducting correlation analyses, we did not see any correlation of neoadjuvant chemo- or radiation therapy with blood loss ($p_{chemo} = 0.977$; $p_{radio} = 0.504$). Correlating the drainage volume to radiation therapy, similarly, showed no statistical significance ($p = 0.800$). When analyzing chemotherapy, however, a significant correlation could be observed with the drainage fluid volume ($p = 0.004$).

4. Discussion

Breast cancer is the most common malignancy in women [40–43]. Although modern diagnostics enable early detection, it often requires mastectomy [44–47]. Thus, breast reconstruction is often needed to prevent the negative after-effects of breast loss [1,48,49]. To facilitate postoperative recovery, paravertebral blocks are used frequently in terms of postoperative pain management [26,29,30,50,51]. This enables early mobilization and shorter hospital stays [33,52,53]. The complications of PVBs are well known and include pneumothorax, pain at the puncture site and dislocation but are generally rare [36–38,54]. However, little is known of their effects on postoperative recovery and blood loss [28,33,52,53].

Nerval blocks are frequently used in replantation surgery, as their vasodilatory effect has proven to be beneficial for limb perfusion [35–39]. This clinical effect suggests that neural blockade interrupts the innervation of vessels, causing vasodilation and thus increasing, e.g., limb perfusion and supporting replantation success. Consequently, it is suspected that paravertebral blocks may also induce vessel dilation and therefore might increase the drainage fluid loss or blood loss. It is assumed that the blockade of sympathetic fibers on vessels sustaining breast perfusion also results in vasodilatory effects, which is made use of in case of limb replantation. Nonetheless, this was not seen in our results. The mean hemoglobin loss did not differ significantly ($p = 0.295$) between groups; moreover, the postoperative hemoglobin levels where similar among our cohort ($p_{postoperative} = 0.604$). Thus, the application of PVB neither led to relevant bleeding at the point of insertion nor at the mastectomy site. Therefore, we can presume that PVB only inhibit nerve fibers that are responsible for pain conduction, which has already been proven by several studies [23–27] (Figure 9).

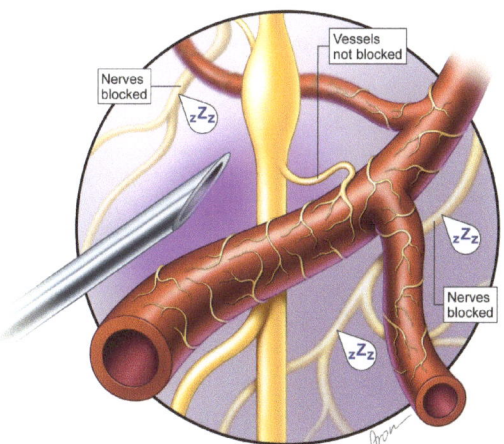

Figure 9. PVB block demonstrating that although pain fibers (marked as "zZz") are blocked, vessel innervation remains unhindered (vessels are not blocked).

The drainage fluid volume was additionally supposed to increase with elevated blood perfusion, as more blood circulation further entails a fluid shift into the extracellular matrix. Nonetheless, this could also not be observed in our study. Here, the postoperative drainage fluid volumes showed no significant difference ($p = 0.508$) and therefore did not lead to delayed drainage removal or prolonged in-hospital treatment.

Overall, women with PVB did not experience any disadvantage in perioperative recovery, as no complications were encountered in relation to paravertebral blocks. Although not quantified, we observed that our patients experienced less pain and tolerated dressing changes better with PVBs installed. These effects of paravertebral blocks are already well known and significantly support breast cancer patients while recovering from surgery [24,26,29,51,55,56]. Consequently, we have implemented the use of paravertebral blocks in our preoperative schedules when planning mastectomies.

However, a few challenges were encountered with PVBs in the daily routine, arising from organizational matters. PVBs require adequately trained anesthesiologists, the coordination of their installation in a specialized setting (ultrasound-guided, trained staff, etc.) and time (approximately 30–60 mins). Also, daily follow-up of proper functionality is required, and early mobilization may sometimes lead to catheter disconnection. Further, a more fundamental insight into the relationship between PVBs and postoperative opioid usage should be achieved in the future.

Additionally, breast cancer staging, as well as hormonal cancer signatures, ought to be addressed in further studies. And although included in our analyses, the relationship between neoadjuvant chemo- and radiation therapy and blood loss and drainage fluid volume is an interesting field of research. Besides chemotherapy appearing to significantly correlate with the drainage fluid volume, unfortunately, this correlation holds diminished value due to its small sample size.

Nevertheless, we consider the usage of paravertebral blocks in post-mastectomy recovery beneficial for our patients. They have been shown to significantly ameliorate patients' postoperative recovery and to reduce the burden put on patients by cancer treatment.

5. Conclusions

Women receiving paravertebral blocks did not experience any disadvantages regarding surgical procedure or postoperative recovery, while early mobilization was possible.

Substantiated by our findings, we recommend including paravertebral blocks in the basic armamentarium when performing mastectomies, as their conduction is safe and feasible.

Author Contributions: Conceptualization, T.F., F.J.J., M.S.M., C.K., C.G., K.P., D.B.L., K.F.S., C.H. and K.D.B.; methodology, T.F., F.J.J., M.S.M., C.K., C.G., K.P., D.B.L., K.F.S., C.H. and K.D.B.; validation, T.F., F.J.J., M.S.M., C.K., C.G., K.P., D.B.L., K.F.S., C.H. and K.D.B.; formal analysis, T.F., F.J.J., M.S.M., C.K., C.G., K.P., D.B.L., K.F.S., C.H. and K.D.B.; investigation, T.F., F.J.J., M.S.M., C.K., C.G., K.P., D.B.L., K.F.S., C.H. and K.D.B.; resources, T.F., F.J.J., M.S.M., C.K., C.G., K.P., D.B.L., K.F.S., C.H. and K.D.B.; data curation, T.F., F.J.J., M.S.M., C.K., C.G., K.P., D.B.L., K.F.S., C.H. and K.D.B.; writing—original draft preparation, T.F., F.J.J., M.S.M., C.K., C.G., K.P., D.B.L., K.F.S., C.H. and K.D.B.; writing—review and editing, T.F., F.J.J., M.S.M., C.K., C.G., K.P., D.B.L., K.F.S., C.H. and K.D.B.; visualization, T.F., F.J.J., M.S.M., C.K., C.G., K.P., D.B.L., K.F.S., C.H. and K.D.B.; supervision, K.F.S., K.D.B.; project administration, T.F.; funding acquisition, T.F. All authors have read and agreed to the published version of the manuscript.

Funding: This research received funding for open access publication from the Karl Landsteiner University of Health Sciences, Dr. Karl-Dorrek-Straße 30, 3500, Krems, Austria.

Institutional Review Board Statement: The study was conducted according to the guidelines of the Declaration of Helsinki and approved by the Institutional Ethics Committee of Karl Landsteiner University of Health Sciences Krems (protocol code: 1085/2023, 10 January 2024).

Informed Consent Statement: Patient consent was waived due to the retrospective character of this study.

Data Availability Statement: All the data analyzed during the current study are available from the corresponding author on reasonable request.

Acknowledgments: The authors want to show appreciation for the contribution of NÖ Landesgesundheitsagentur, the legal entity of University Hospitals in Lower Austria, for providing the organizational framework to conduct this research. The authors would also like to acknowledge support from the Open Access Publishing Fund of Karl Landsteiner University of Health Sciences, Krems, Austria. This work was supported by Forschungsimpulse [project ID: SF_61], a program of Karl Landsteiner University of Health Sciences, funded by the Federal Government of Lower Austria. We also thank Aron Cserveny for providing the graphics. We received Open Access Funding by Karl Landsteiner University of Health Sciences, Krems, Austria.

Conflicts of Interest: The authors declare no conflicts of interest.

References

1. Bergmeister, K.D.; Rohrbacher, A.; Flores, T.; Bachner, M.G.; Gotzinger, P.; Schrogendorfer, K.F. Breast reconstruction following cancer. *Wien. Klin. Wochenschr.* **2020**, *132*, 475–489. [CrossRef] [PubMed]
2. Zhang, C.; Kosiorek, H.; Hammond, J.B.; Jogerst, K.M.; Cronin, P.; Ahmad, S.; Rebecca, A.; Casey, W.; Pockaj, B.A. The impact of mastectomy and reconstruction technique on patient perceived quality of Life. *Am. J. Surg.* **2022**, *224*, 1450–1454. [CrossRef] [PubMed]
3. Kiebert, G.M.; de Haes, J.C.; van de Velde, C.J. The impact of breast-conserving treatment and mastectomy on the quality of life of early-stage breast cancer patients: A review. *J. Clin. Oncol.* **1991**, *9*, 1059–1070. [CrossRef] [PubMed]
4. Kakati, B.; Nair, N.; Chatterjee, A. Post mastectomy pain syndrome at an Indian tertiary cancer centre and its impact on quality of life. *Indian J. Cancer* **2023**, *60*, 275–281. [CrossRef]
5. Dinapoli, L.; Colloca, G.; Di Capua, B.; Valentini, V. Psychological Aspects to Consider in Breast Cancer Diagnosis and Treatment. *Curr. Oncol. Rep.* **2021**, *23*, 38. [CrossRef]
6. Hanson, S.E.; Lei, X.; Roubaud, M.S.; DeSnyder, S.M.; Caudle, A.S.; Shaitelman, S.F.; Hoffman, K.E.; Smith, G.L.; Jagsi, R.; Peterson, S.K.; et al. Long-Term Quality of Life in Patients with Breast Cancer After Breast Conservation vs Mastectomy and Reconstruction. *JAMA Surg.* **2022**, *157*, e220631. [CrossRef]
7. Zehra, S.; Doyle, F.; Barry, M.; Walsh, S.; Kell, M.R. Health-related quality of life following breast reconstruction compared to total mastectomy and breast-conserving surgery among breast cancer survivors: A systematic review and meta-analysis. *Breast Cancer* **2020**, *27*, 534–566. [CrossRef]

8. Victoria, M.; Marie, B.; Dominique, R.; Caroline, A.; Marc-Karim, B.D.; Julien, M.; Sophie, L.; Anne-Deborah, B. Breast reconstruction and quality of life five years after cancer diagnosis: VICAN French National cohort. *Breast Cancer Res. Treat.* **2022**, *194*, 449–461. [CrossRef]
9. Ginsburg, O.; Bray, F.; Coleman, M.P.; Vanderpuye, V.; Eniu, A.; Kotha, S.R.; Sarker, M.; Huong, T.T.; Allemani, C.; Dvaladze, A.; et al. The global burden of women's cancers: A grand challenge in global health. *Lancet* **2017**, *389*, 847–860. [CrossRef]
10. Moo, T.A.; Nelson, J.A.; Sevilimedu, V.; Charyn, J.; Le, T.V.; Allen, R.J.; Mehrara, B.J.; Barrio, A.V.; Capko, D.M.; Pilewskie, M.; et al. Strategies to avoid mastectomy skin-flap necrosis during nipple-sparing mastectomy. *Br. J. Surg.* **2023**, *110*, 831–838. [CrossRef]
11. Galimberti, V.; Vicini, E.; Corso, G.; Morigi, C.; Fontana, S.; Sacchini, V.; Veronesi, P. Nipple-sparing and skin-sparing mastectomy: Review of aims, oncological safety and contraindications. *Breast* **2017**, *34* (Suppl. S1), S82–S84. [CrossRef] [PubMed]
12. Pagliara, D.; Schiavone, L.; Garganese, G.; Bove, S.; Montella, R.A.; Costantini, M.; Rinaldi, P.M.; Bottosso, S.; Grieco, F.; Rubino, C.; et al. Predicting Mastectomy Skin Flap Necrosis: A Systematic Review of Preoperative and Intraoperative Assessment Techniques. *Clin. Breast Cancer* **2023**, *23*, 249–254. [CrossRef] [PubMed]
13. Tang, N.; Li, H.; Chow, Y.; Blake, W. Non-operative adjuncts for the prevention of mastectomy skin flap necrosis: A systematic review and meta-analysis. *ANZ J. Surg.* **2023**, *93*, 65–75. [CrossRef] [PubMed]
14. Oleck, N.C.; Gu, C.; Pyfer, B.J.; Phillips, B.T. Defining Mastectomy Skin Flap Necrosis: A Systematic Review of the Literature and a Call for Standardization. *Plast. Reconstr. Surg.* **2022**, *149*, 858e–866e. [CrossRef]
15. Matsen, C.B.; Mehrara, B.; Eaton, A.; Capko, D.; Berg, A.; Stempel, M.; Van Zee, K.J.; Pusic, A.; King, T.A.; Cody, H.S., 3rd; et al. Skin Flap Necrosis After Mastectomy with Reconstruction: A Prospective Study. *Ann. Surg. Oncol.* **2016**, *23*, 257–264. [CrossRef]
16. Dawson, S.E.; Berns, J.M.; Tran, P.C.; Fisher, C.S.; Ludwig, K.K.; Lester, M.E.; Hassanein, A.H. Optimizing tissue expander breast reconstruction in nicotine users: An algorithmic approach. *J. Plast. Reconstr. Aesthet. Surg.* **2022**, *75*, 3628–3651. [CrossRef]
17. Soni, S.E.; Le, N.K.; Buller, M.; Modica, A.D.; Kumar, A.; Smith, P.D.; Laronga, C. Complication Profile of Total Submuscular Versus Prepectoral Tissue Expander Placement: A Retrospective Cohort Study. *Ann. Plast. Surg.* **2022**, *88*, S439–S442. [CrossRef]
18. Payne, S.H.; Ballesteros, S.; Brown, O.H.; Razavi, S.A.; Carlson, G.W. Skin Reducing Mastectomy and Immediate Tissue Expander Reconstruction: A Critical Analysis. *Ann. Plast. Surg.* **2022**, *88*, 485–489. [CrossRef]
19. Leiman, D.; Barlow, M.; Carpin, K.; Pina, E.M.; Casso, D. Medial and lateral pectoral nerve block with liposomal bupivacaine for the management of postsurgical pain after submuscular breast augmentation. *Plast. Reconstr. Surg. Glob. Open* **2014**, *2*, e282. [CrossRef]
20. Hagarty, S.E.; Yen, L.L.; Luo, J.; Fosco, C.R.; Gomez, K.; Khare, M. Decreased Length of Postoperative Drain Use, Parenteral Opioids, Length of Stay, and Complication Rates in Patients Receiving Meshed versus Unmeshed Acellular Dermal Matrix in 194 Submuscular Tissue Expander-Based Breast Reconstructions: A Single-Surgeon Cohort Study. *Plast. Reconstr. Surg.* **2020**, *145*, 889–897. [CrossRef]
21. Zhu, L.; Mohan, A.T.; Abdelsattar, J.M.; Wang, Z.; Vijayasekaran, A.; Hwang, S.M.; Tran, N.V.; Saint-Cyr, M. Comparison of subcutaneous versus submuscular expander placement in the first stage of immediate breast reconstruction. *J. Plast. Reconstr. Aesthet. Surg.* **2016**, *69*, e77–e86. [CrossRef]
22. Cattelani, L.; Polotto, S.; Arcuri, M.F.; Pedrazzi, G.; Linguadoca, C.; Bonati, E. One-Step Prepectoral Breast Reconstruction with Dermal Matrix-Covered Implant Compared to Submuscular Implantation: Functional and Cost Evaluation. *Clin. Breast Cancer* **2018**, *18*, e703–e711. [CrossRef] [PubMed]
23. Albi-Feldzer, A.; Dureau, S.; Ghimouz, A.; Raft, J.; Soubirou, J.L.; Gayraud, G.; Jayr, C. Preoperative Paravertebral Block and Chronic Pain After Breast Cancer Surgery: A Double-Blind Randomized Trial. *Anesthesiology* **2021**, *135*, 1091–1103. [CrossRef] [PubMed]
24. Buzney, C.D.; Lin, L.Z.; Chatterjee, A.; Gallagher, S.W.; Quraishi, S.A.; Drzymalski, D.M. Association Between Paravertebral Block and Pain Score at the Time of Hospital Discharge in Oncoplastic Breast Surgery: A Retrospective Cohort Study. *Plast. Reconstr. Surg.* **2021**, *147*, 928e–935e. [CrossRef]
25. Rawal, N. Current issues in postoperative pain management. *Eur. J. Anaesthesiol.* **2016**, *33*, 160–171. [CrossRef]
26. Sivrikoz, N.; Turhan, O.; Ali, A.; Altun, D.; Tukenmez, M.; Sungur, Z. Paravertebral block versus erector spinae plane block for analgesia in modified radical mastectomy: A randomized, prospective, double-blind study. *Minerva Anestesiol.* **2022**, *88*, 1003–1012. [CrossRef]
27. Xiong, C.; Han, C.; Zhao, D.; Peng, W.; Xu, D.; Lan, Z. Postoperative analgesic effects of paravertebral block versus erector spinae plane block for thoracic and breast surgery: A meta-analysis. *PLoS ONE* **2021**, *16*, e0256611. [CrossRef]
28. Vila, H., Jr.; Liu, J.; Kavasmaneck, D. Paravertebral block: New benefits from an old procedure. *Curr. Opin. Anaesthesiol.* **2007**, *20*, 316–318. [CrossRef]
29. Heesen, M.; Klimek, M.; Rossaint, R.; Imberger, G.; Straube, S. Paravertebral block and persistent postoperative pain after breast surgery: Meta-analysis and trial sequential analysis. *Anaesthesia* **2016**, *71*, 1471–1481. [CrossRef]
30. Yeung, J.H.; Gates, S.; Naidu, B.V.; Wilson, M.J.; Gao Smith, F. Paravertebral block versus thoracic epidural for patients undergoing thoracotomy. *Cochrane Database Syst. Rev.* **2016**, *2*, CD009121. [CrossRef]

31. Niesen, A.D.; Jacob, A.K.; Law, L.A.; Sviggum, H.P.; Johnson, R.L. Complication rate of ultrasound-guided paravertebral block for breast surgery. *Reg. Anesth. Pain Med.* **2020**, *45*, 813–817. [CrossRef] [PubMed]
32. Ardon, A.E.; Lee, J.; Franco, C.D.; Riutort, K.T.; Greengrass, R.A. Paravertebral block: Anatomy and relevant safety issues. *Korean J. Anesthesiol.* **2020**, *73*, 394–400. [CrossRef] [PubMed]
33. Slinchenkova, K.; Lee, K.; Choudhury, S.; Sundarapandiyan, D.; Gritsenko, K. A Review of the Paravertebral Block: Benefits and Complications. *Curr. Pain Headache Rep.* **2023**, *27*, 203–208. [CrossRef]
34. Ardon, A.E.; Curley, E.; Greengrass, R. Safety and Complications of Landmark-Based Paravertebral Blocks: A Retrospective Analysis of 979 Patients and 4983 Injections. *Clin. J. Pain* **2024**, *40*, 367–372. [CrossRef]
35. Kim, M.K.; Yi, M.S.; Park, P.G.; Kang, H.; Lee, J.S.; Shin, H.Y. Effect of Stellate Ganglion Block on the Regional Hemodynamics of the Upper Extremity: A Randomized Controlled Trial. *Anesth. Analg.* **2018**, *126*, 1705–1711. [CrossRef]
36. Kim, J.; Park, K.; Cho, Y.; Lee, J. The Effects of Vasodilation Induced by Brachial Plexus Block on the Development of Postoperative Thrombosis of the Arteriovenous Access in Patients with End-Stage Renal Disease: A Retrospective Study. *Int. J. Environ. Res. Public Health* **2022**, *19*, 5158. [CrossRef]
37. Bas, S.; Hascicek, S.; Ucak, R.; Gunenc, A.; Yesilada, A.K. Effect of perivascular low dose ethanol on rat femoral vessels: Preliminary study. *J. Plast. Surg. Hand Surg.* **2020**, *54*, 358–364. [CrossRef]
38. Cayci, C.; Cinar, C.; Yucel, O.A.; Tekinay, T.; Ascherman, J.A. The effect of epidural anesthesia on muscle flap tolerance to venous ischemia. *Plast. Reconstr. Surg.* **2010**, *125*, 89–98. [CrossRef]
39. Flores, T.; Jaklin, F.J.; Rohrbacher, A.; Schrogendorfer, K.F.; Bergmeister, K.D. Perioperative Risk Factors for Prolonged Blood Loss and Drainage Fluid Secretion after Breast Reconstruction. *J. Clin. Med.* **2022**, *11*, 808. [CrossRef]
40. Merino Bonilla, J.A.; Torres Tabanera, M.; Ros Mendoza, L.H. Breast cancer in the 21st century: From early detection to new therapies. *Radiologia* **2017**, *59*, 368–379. [CrossRef]
41. Cardoso, F.; Kyriakides, S.; Ohno, S.; Penault-Llorca, F.; Poortmans, P.; Rubio, I.T.; Zackrisson, S.; Senkus, E.; ESMO Guidelines Committee. Early breast cancer: ESMO Clinical Practice Guidelines for diagnosis, treatment and follow-updagger. *Ann. Oncol.* **2019**, *30*, 1194–1220. [CrossRef] [PubMed]
42. Abo Al-Shiekh, S.S.; Ibrahim, M.A.; Alajerami, Y.S. Breast Cancer Knowledge and Practice of Breast Self-Examination among Female University Students, Gaza. *Sci. World J.* **2021**, *2021*, 6640324. [CrossRef] [PubMed]
43. Rahman, W.T.; Helvie, M.A. Breast cancer screening in average and high-risk women. *Best Pract. Res. Clin. Obstet. Gynaecol.* **2022**, *83*, 3–14. [CrossRef]
44. Heemskerk-Gerritsen, B.A.; Brekelmans, C.T.; Menke-Pluymers, M.B.; van Geel, A.N.; Tilanus-Linthorst, M.M.; Bartels, C.C.; Tan, M.; Meijers-Heijboer, H.E.; Klijn, J.G.; Seynaeve, C. Prophylactic mastectomy in BRCA1/2 mutation carriers and women at risk of hereditary breast cancer: Long-term experiences at the Rotterdam Family Cancer Clinic. *Ann. Surg. Oncol.* **2007**, *14*, 3335–3344. [CrossRef]
45. Henry, D.A.; Lee, M.C.; Almanza, D.; Ahmed, K.A.; Sun, W.; Boulware, D.C.; Laronga, C. Trends in use of bilateral prophylactic mastectomy vs high-risk surveillance in unaffected carriers of inherited breast cancer syndromes in the Inherited Cancer Registry (ICARE). *Breast Cancer Res. Treat.* **2019**, *174*, 39–45. [CrossRef]
46. Wong, S.M.; Apostolova, C.; Eisenberg, E.; Foulkes, W.D. Counselling Framework for Germline BRCA1/2 and PALB2 Carriers Considering Risk-Reducing Mastectomy. *Curr. Oncol.* **2024**, *31*, 350–365. [CrossRef]
47. Qin, R.; Yin, L.; Wang, D.; Cao, X.; Shaibu, Z.; Wang, X.; Chen, P.; Sui, D.; Qiu, X.; Liu, D. Survival Outcomes of Breast-Conserving Surgery Versus Mastectomy in Locally Advanced Breast Cancer Following Neoadjuvant Chemotherapy: A Meta-Analysis. *Technol. Cancer Res. Treat.* **2024**, *23*, 15330338241265030. [CrossRef]
48. Bolliger, M.; Gambone, L.; Haeusler, T.; Mikula, F.; Kampf, S.; Fitzal, F. Patient Satisfaction, Esthetic Outcome, and Quality of Life in Oncoplastic and Reconstructive Breast Surgery: A Single Center Experience. *Breast Care* **2024**, *19*, 215–222. [CrossRef]
49. Mustata, L.M.; Peltecu, G.; Gica, N.; Botezatu, R.; Iancu, G.; Gheoca, G.D.; Cigaran, R.; Iordachescu, D.A. Evaluation of quality of life and socio-emotional impact of oncological treatment among patients with breast cancer. *J. Med. Life* **2024**, *17*, 341–352. [CrossRef]
50. Plunkett, A.; Scott, T.L.; Tracy, E. Regional anesthesia for breast cancer surgery: Which block is best? A review of the current literature. *Pain Manag.* **2022**, *12*, 943–950. [CrossRef]
51. Grape, S.; El-Boghdadly, K.; Albrecht, E. Analgesic efficacy of PECS vs paravertebral blocks after radical mastectomy: A systematic review, meta-analysis and trial sequential analysis. *J. Clin. Anesth.* **2020**, *63*, 109745. [CrossRef] [PubMed]
52. Mishra, N.; Haque, E.; Bhagat, M.; Kumar, V.; Suwalka, U.; Gorai, P. Use of Paravertebral Block as an Alternative to General Anesthesia for Breast Surgeries: A Randomized Control Study. *Cureus* **2021**, *13*, e18322. [CrossRef] [PubMed]
53. Fei, M.; Qin, W.; An, G.; Li, D.; Li, C.; Xiong, L. Comparison of paravertebral block vs. general anesthesia for percutaneous nephrolithotomy: A retrospective study. *Front. Med.* **2023**, *10*, 1081530. [CrossRef] [PubMed]
54. Tsuneyoshi, I.; Onomoto, M.; Yonetani, A.; Kanmura, Y. Low-dose vasopressin infusion in patients with severe vasodilatory hypotension after prolonged hemorrhage during general anesthesia. *J. Anesth.* **2005**, *19*, 170–173. [CrossRef]

55. But, M.; Wernicki, K.; Zielinski, J.; Szczecinska, W. A Comparison of the Effectiveness of the Serratus Anterior Plane Block and Erector Spinae Plane Block to that of the Paravertebral Block in the Surgical Treatment of Breast Cancer—A Randomized, Prospective, Single-Blinded Study. *J. Clin. Med.* **2024**, *13*, 4836. [CrossRef]
56. Chappell, A.G.; Yuksel, S.; Sasson, D.C.; Wescott, A.B.; Connor, L.M.; Ellis, M.F. Post-Mastectomy Pain Syndrome: An Up-to-Date Review of Treatment Outcomes. *JPRAS Open* **2021**, *30*, 97–109. [CrossRef]

Disclaimer/Publisher's Note: The statements, opinions and data contained in all publications are solely those of the individual author(s) and contributor(s) and not of MDPI and/or the editor(s). MDPI and/or the editor(s) disclaim responsibility for any injury to people or property resulting from any ideas, methods, instructions or products referred to in the content.

MDPI AG
Grosspeteranlage 5
4052 Basel
Switzerland
Tel.: +41 61 683 77 34

Journal of Clinical Medicine Editorial Office
E-mail: jcm@mdpi.com
www.mdpi.com/journal/jcm

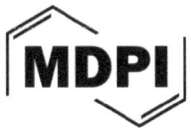

Disclaimer/Publisher's Note: The title and front matter of this reprint are at the discretion of the Guest Editors. The publisher is not responsible for their content or any associated concerns. The statements, opinions and data contained in all individual articles are solely those of the individual Editors and contributors and not of MDPI. MDPI disclaims responsibility for any injury to people or property resulting from any ideas, methods, instructions or products referred to in the content.

www.ingramcontent.com/pod-product-compliance
Lightning Source LLC
LaVergne TN
LVHW070000100526
838202LV00019B/2590